E.I. Hernández-Jiménez

CELLULITE, LOCALIZED FAT DEPOSITS, AND BODY CONTOURING

IN COSMETIC DERMATOLOGY & SKINCARE PRACTICE

Cosmetics & Medicine
Publishing

Author/Editor:
Elena I. Hernández-Jiménez, *Ph.D.*

CELLULITE, LOCALIZED FAT DEPOSITS, AND BODY CONTOURING IN COSMETIC DERMATOLOGY AND SKINCARE PRACTICE

This book is a practice-oriented resource grounded in current scientific knowledge and evidence-based aesthetic practice, focused on cellulite, localized fat deposits, and body contouring. It integrates core concepts in skin biology with detailed, clinically relevant overviews of remodeling technologies used in aesthetics.

The opening chapters provide essential background on the structure and physiology of SAT, the pathways of lipogenesis and lipolysis, key differences among adipocyte populations, contributing factors in cellulite, and skin changes associated with excess weight. This foundation clarifies the biological targets for intervention and supports sound selection of treatment approaches.

The core chapters focus on scientifically supported approaches to reducing fat deposits, improving skin firmness, and enhancing body contours. They cover:

- Technology-based care: Mechanotherapy (massage, pressotherapy, vibrotherapy, vacuum techniques), electrotherapy (microcurrents, electric myostimulation, magnetic myostimulation, radiofrequency therapy), ultrasound cavitation, high-intensity focused ultrasound, shockwave therapy, laser lipolysis, and cryolipolysis.
- Injectables: Physiologic stimulation of lipolysis, lipodestruction, mesotherapy, collagen therapy, and carboxytherapy.
- Topical care: Active ingredients aimed at lipolysis, dermal-matrix support, and edema reduction, along with professional procedures (thalassotherapy, mud therapy, wraps).
- Additional tools: Nutraceuticals, weight-management medications, and specialized compression garments.

A dedicated chapter addresses how to choose the most appropriate procedure — or combination of methods — based on cellulite stage, skin condition, and overall health status. The author explains the mechanisms behind each technology, along with clinical effects, indications, contraindications, potential risks, and practical criteria for evaluating results.

This book will help you:

- Deepen your understanding of the biological basis of cellulite and localized fat deposits.
- Select appropriate interventions for different clinical situations.
- Build comprehensive body-contouring programs.
- Explain to patients the real possibilities and limitations of procedures.
- Improve the quality and effectiveness of day-to-day practice.

This publication is intended for aesthetic practitioners, skincare professionals, and massage therapists, as well as students in skincare and massage training programs — and anyone who wants a more profound, practice-focused understanding of modern body-contouring approaches.

ISBN 978-1-970196-51-1 (paperback)
ISBN 978-1-970196-52-8 (hardcover)
ISBN 978-1-970196-53-5 (eBook – Adobe PDF)
ISBN 978-1-970196-54-2 (eBook – ePUB)

Translated and edited by the author with AI assistance.

Author/Editor

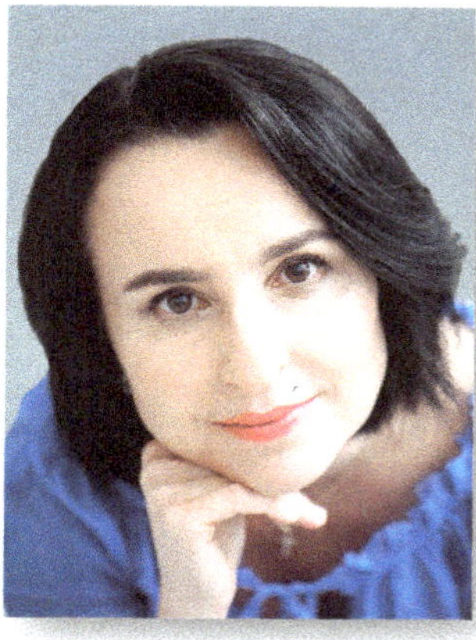

Elena I. Hernández-Jiménez, *Ph.D.*

Biophysicist, scientific journalist

Editor-in-chief of Cosmetics and Medicine Publishing

Member of the International Society of Applied Corneotherapy (I.A.C.); Chair of the I.A.C. Executive Board (May, 2019 – May, 2025)

Author and co-author of numerous publications in professional magazines, co-author and editor of the book series *Fundamentals of Cosmetic Dermatology & Skincare*, *Cosmetic Dermatology & Skincare Practice*, *Cosmetic Chemistry for Dermatology & Skincare Specialists* and others

Speaker at international conferences, author of training seminars and webinars for professionals in the field of skincare

Professional interests: biology and physiology of the skin, skin permeability, cosmetic chemistry, anti-age medicine, physiotherapy in dermatology and aesthetic medicine, skin analysis and imaging

Table of Contents

List of abbreviations 10
Introduction 12

PART I
BIOLOGY AND PHYSIOLOGY OF ADIPOSE TISSUE

Chapter 1. Subcutaneous adipose tissue 14
1.1. Body fat depots 14
1.2. Adipocyte: the primary cell of adipose tissue 15
1.2.1. Origin 16
1.2.2. Types of adipocytes 18
White adipocytes 18
Brown adipocytes 19
Beige adipocytes 19
Pink adipocytes 19
Yellow adipocytes 20
1.2.3. Distribution of adipocytes 20
1.3. Fat metabolism 22
1.3.1. Triglycerides: the primary component of fat 22
1.3.2. Lipogenesis and lipolysis: the two sides of fat metabolism 23
1.4. Other cells of adipose tissue 24
1.5. Adipose tissue as an endocrine organ 26
1.6. Aging of adipose tissue 26
1.7. Aesthetic problems related and not related to SAT 27

Chapter 2. Cellulite 29
2.1. Causes of cellulite 30
2.2. Stages and symptoms 32

Chapter 3. Obesity: What to expect in the skin? **34**
3.1. Skin pathophysiology in obesity 36
3.1.1. Skin barrier 36
3.1.2. Sebaceous glands 37
3.1.3. Sweat glands 37
3.1.4. Collagen and wound healing 38
3.1.5. Microcirculatory bed 38
3.2. Obesity and skin diseases 38
3.2.1. Dermatoses 40
3.2.2. Skin infections 40
3.2.3. Metabolic disorders 42
3.3. Common skin manifestations in obesity 42
3.4. Obesity and rare skin conditions 43

PART II

COMMON APPROACHES TO SUBCUTANEOUS ADIPOSE TISSUE REMODELING

1.1. Scientific substantiation of lipolysis-stimulating strategies 48
1.2. SAT-targeted modalities 51
1.3. Selecting interventions based on the stage of cellulite 53
Stage 1 53
Stage 2 54
Stage 3 54
Stage 4 55

PART III

LIPOSUCTION

1.1. Suction-assisted lipectomy (aspiration liposuction) 57
1.2. Vibration-assisted liposuction (booster liposuction) 58
1.3. Radiofrequency-assisted liposuction 58
1.4. Laser-assisted liposuction 60
1.5. Ultrasound-assisted liposuction 60
1.6. Treatment of post-liposuction skin irregularities 61

PART IV

BODY-CONTOURING DEVICES AND PROCEDURES

Chapter 1. Mechanical technologies **65**

1.1. Mechanotherapy: molecular and cellular mechanisms 66

1.1.1. Cell cytoskeleton and extracellular matrix 67

1.1.2. PIEZO channels: cellular mechanoreceptors 68

1.1.3. Tactile receptors: mechanoreceptors of the skin 69

1.2. Mechanotherapy technologies: variants and effects 72

1.2.1. Manual massage 72

1.2.2. Compression therapy 73

Pressotherapy 73

Shiatsu massage 74

1.2.3. Vibration therapy 75

1.2.4. Vacuum therapy (decompression) 76

1.3. Combined mechanotherapy 77

1.3.1. Vibrovacuum therapy: decompression + vibration 77

1.3.2. Vacuum-roller massage: decompression + kneading 78

1.3.3. Vibrocompression therapy 79

1.4. Future for mechanotherapy 81

Chapter 2. Electrical technologies **83**

2.1. Basic characteristics of electric current 83

2.2. Interaction of electric current and biological tissue 86

2.2.1. Tissue conductivity 86

2.2.2. Thermal effects of electric current 87

Direct and low-frequency currents 87

High-frequency currents 88

2.2.3. Non-thermal effects of electric current 88

2.3. Electrotherapy technologies: variants and effects 89

2.3.1. Resistive technologies 89

Monopolar devices 90

Bipolar devices 91

Multipolar devices 92

2.3.2. Capacitive technologies 92

2.3.3. Inductive technologies 93

2.4. High-frequency therapy 94

2.4.1. Radiofrequency therapy (RF therapy) 94
RF-assisted liposuction 96
RF-assisted lipolysis 97
RF diathermy and electroporation 99
RF microneedling 100
2.4.2. Ultra-high frequency therapy (UHF therapy) 101
UHF therapy effects 102
UHF technologies 104
2.5. Electrolipolysis 106
2.6. Neuromuscular stimulation 108
2.6.1. Physiology of neuromuscular stimulation 111
2.6.2. Neuromuscular stimulation technologies: variants and effects 111
Current distribution with depth 112
Subjective sensations during the procedure 113
Guidelines for technology selection 113
2.6.3. Magnetic myostimulation 114
2.6.4. Electromyostimulation 116
2.7. Microcurrent therapy 117
2.8. Gel for electrotherapy procedures 119
Chapter 3. Sound technologies 121
3.1. Ultrasound therapy 121
3.1.1 Ultrasonic cavitation (low-frequency ultrasound) 122
Focused vs. non-focused delivery 123
3.1.2. Ultrasonic thermocoagulation (high-frequency ultrasound) 125
3.2. Extracorporeal shockwave therapy 128
3.2.1. Shockwave effects on SAT 128
3.2.2. Radial and focused shockwave therapy 130
3.2.3. Shockwave therapy in complex anti-cellulite programs ... 132
3.3. Gel for ultrasound and shockwave treatments 133
Chapter 4. Light technologies 135
4.1. Interaction of light with biological tissues 135
4.2. Laser lipolysis as an alternative to traditional liposuction 136
4.3. Laser lipolysis technologies: variants and effects 137

4.3.1. "Hot" laser lipolysis 137
Minimally invasive laser lipolysis and laser-assisted liposuction 139
Non-invasive laser lipolysis 140
4.3.2 "Cold" laser lipolysis 141
Chapter 5. Cryolipolysis 143
5.1. Historical background 143
5.2. Cryolipolysis technologies: variants and effects 145
5.2.1. Vacuum-assisted cryolipolysis 145
5.2.2. Contrast cryolipolysis 151
5.2.3 Cryolipolysis with plates 153
5.2.4. Electromyostimulation + cooling 153
5.3. Indications and contraindications 154
5.4. Factors affecting efficacy 155
5.4.1. Patient selection 156
5.4.2. Technical issues 156
Volume of cooled adipose tissue 156
Temperature in the exposure zone 157
Session duration 158
Number of treatments 158
Mechanical effects 158
5.5. Procedure 159
5.6. Undesirable phenomena and complications 160
5.6.1. Post-session reactions and complications 160
5.6.2. Paradoxical adipose hyperplasia 160
Frequency of occurrence 160
Causes 162
Risk factors 164
Chapter 6. Combined technologies 166

PART V
INJECTION TREATMENT
1.1. Improvement of microcirculation 170
1.2. Impact on adipose tissue 171

1.2.1. Physiologic regulation of lipolysis 171
1.2.2. Lipodestruction 176
Fat emulsification ("fat dissolution") 176
Hypotonic destruction of adipocytes 182
Injectable cryolipolysis 183
1.3. Skin thickening 185
1.3.1. Mesotherapy 185
1.3.2. Collagen therapy 186
1.4. Carboxytherapy 187

PART VI
ANTI-CELLULITE COSMETIC PRODUCTS
1.1. Active ingredients 193
1.1.1. Stimulation of lipolysis 193
1.1.2. Fat burning 193
1.1.3. Strengthening the collagen–elastin framework and improving the dermal structure 194
1.1.4 Reduction of edema, improvement of microcirculation ... 194
1.1.5. Anti-cellulite complexes 194
1.2. Professional cosmetic treatments 196
1.2.1. Thalassotherapy 196
1.2.2. Mud therapy 196
1.2.3. Wraps 197

PART VII
OTHER METHODS FOR BODY CONTOURING
1.1. Nutraceuticals 199
1.2. Drugs for blood sugar control and weight loss 200
1.3. Specialized clothing 202

Conclusion 203
References 204

List of abbreviations

ADSCs — adipose tissue-derived stem cells
AMPK — AMP-activated protein kinase
ATP — adenosine triphosphate
BDNF — brain-derived neurotrophic factor
BMI — body mass index
BMP — bone morphogenetic protein
CaHA — calcium hydroxyapatite
cAMP — cyclic adenosine monophosphate
CCL2 — C-C motif chemokine ligand 2
CNS — central nervous system
CTGF — connective tissue growth factor
CYR61 — cysteine-rich angiogenic inducer 61
DC — sodium deoxycholate
DGL — diglyceride lipase
DPP-4 — dipeptidyl peptidase-4
EMS — electromyostimulation
FDA — U.S. Food and Drug Administration
FFA — free fatty acids
FGF — fibroblast growth factor
FSTL1 — follistatin-like protein 1
GLP-1 — glucagon-like peptide-1
HDL — high-density lipoprotein
HGH — human growth hormone (somatotropin)
HIFEM — high-intensity focused electromagnetic energy
HIFU — high-intensity focused ultrasound
IGF-1 — insulin-like growth factor 1
IL — interleukin
IPL — intense pulsed light
LDL — low-density lipoprotein
LIF — leukemia inhibitory factor
LLLI — low-level laser irradiation
LLLT — low-level laser (light) therapy
MGL — monoglyceride lipase
MMP — matrix metalloproteinase
MRI — magnetic resonance imaging
MSCs — mesenchymal stem cells

Nd:YAG — neodymium-doped yttrium aluminum garnet
PAH — paradoxical adipose hyperplasia
PC — phosphatidylcholine
PGC1 — peroxisome proliferator-activated receptor-coactivator 1
PPARγ — peroxisome proliferator-activated receptor gamma
RF — radiofrequency
RFAL — radiofrequency-assisted liposuction
ROS — reactive oxygen species
SAT — subcutaneous adipose tissue
SMAS — superficial musculoaponeurotic system
SVF — stromal vascular fraction
TEWL — transepidermal water loss
TGF-β — transforming growth factor beta
TGL — triglyceride lipase
TNF-α — tumor necrosis factor alpha
UCP1 — uncoupling protein 1
UHF — ultra-high frequency
VAS — Visual Analog Scale
VEGF — vascular endothelial growth factor

Introduction

Body contouring is one of the most common requests in modern aesthetic medicine. It is a complex task, with solutions depending on various factors. The shape of our body is formed by different anatomical structures at varying depths. Their configuration is primarily determined by genetics, but an individual's lifestyle can lead to significant alterations. Different specialists focus on specific structures: orthopedists and traumatologists address the musculoskeletal system, endocrinologists and nutritionists manage visceral fat, and physical therapists and massage therapists work with the ligamentous and muscular stabilizing systems. Skincare professionals concentrate on the skin and subcutaneous tissues.

This book explores how changes in these tissues affect body contours and describes the aesthetic methods to influence body shape when clients seek their expertise.

Part I

Biology and physiology of adipose tissue

Chapter 1
Subcutaneous adipose tissue

Body contours are shaped mainly by the amount and distribution of body fat. For that reason, adipose tissue sits at the center of most body contouring work and is the primary focus of this book.

1.1. Body fat depots

In humans, adipose tissue is found in several anatomical zones:

- **Subcutaneous adipose tissue (SAT)** is a dense fat layer located directly beneath the skin, which is why it is also referred to as the hypodermis.
- **Visceral fat** is a relatively loose form of adipose tissue located in the abdominal cavity, surrounding internal organs such as the liver, pancreas, and intestines.
- **Bone marrow adipose tissue** is found in the medullary canals of tubular bones and within the cellular spaces of cancellous bone.
- **Mammary adipose tissue** is located beneath the skin and within the mammary gland itself, between the lobes.

Adipose tissue in each zone has distinct properties. **Only the SAT is readily accessible for aesthetic intervention.** At the same time, some device-based technologies have been shown to influence visceral fat, which supports their use in weight-management programs.

The SAT consists of two layers separated by a connective tissue plane (**Fig. I-1-1**). The upper layer, which lies directly adjacent to the dermis, contains large, round fat cells embedded in a fibrous network with vertically oriented septa. Numerous small vessels run between

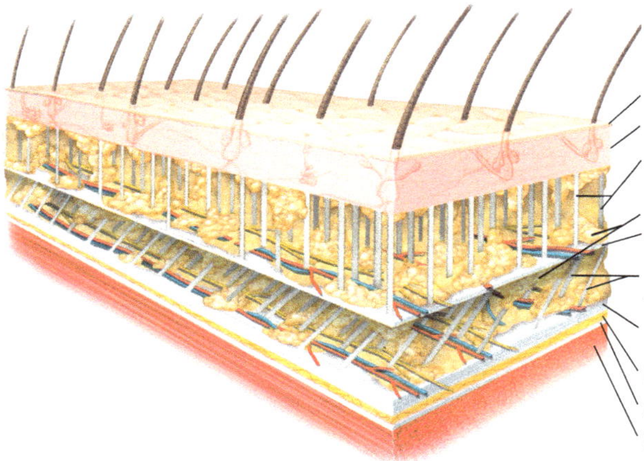

Fig. I-1-1. Schematic illustration of skin and SAT architecture (adapted from Celik N. et al., 2018; CC BY)

the cells. In women and children, this layer is typically thicker than in men. The lower layer contains smaller cells embedded in a fibrous matrix with horizontally oriented septa and is associated with larger vessels. With weight gain, the number of cells in this layer increases (Celik N. et al., 2018).

Beyond structural differences, adipose tissue from different regions also varies in adipocyte composition. Let's take a closer look.

1.2. Adipocyte: the primary cell of adipose tissue

Adipocytes are the key cells of adipose tissue. They store and process lipids and produce hormones that regulate energy metabolism. Importantly, adipose tissue begins forming early in life. The number of adipocytes increases until roughly 20 years of age and then generally stabilizes.

After that point, the number of fat cells may still increase under certain conditions, but it typically does not decrease.

Total adipose-tissue volume depends not only on the number of adipocytes but also on their size: people with obesity tend to have larger adipocytes than lean individuals. A few clinically relevant reference points:

- **Cell number:** Lean individuals have fewer fat cells than individuals with obesity (30×10^9 vs. $80–100 \times 10^9$).
- **Cell size**: Adipocyte diameter ranges from 20 to 180 μm and can shift over time; in some cases, small adipocytes enlarge up to their maximal size.

1.2.1. Origin

Adipocytes originate from **mesenchymal stem cells (MSCs)**, which reside in the mesenchyme — the connective tissue present within many organs and tissues. MSCs can differentiate into multiple specialized lineages, including osteocytes, chondrocytes, myocytes, stromal cells, fibroblasts, neurons, and adipocytes.

MSCs differentiation into adipocytes proceeds through several stages (**Fig. I-1-2**). First, MSCs give rise to proliferating preadipocytes — precursor cells that can both multiply and begin accumulating lipids. As maturation continues, preadipocytes acquire hallmark adipocyte features: they intensify lipid synthesis, form intracellular lipid droplets, and express adipocyte-associated markers such as perilipin (a protein that coats lipid droplets in white adipocytes) and uncoupling protein 1 (UCP1; thermogenin), a mitochondrial carrier protein characteristic of brown adipose tissue). With continued growth and differentiation, these precursors become fully functional adipocytes capable of energy storage and endocrine activity (Obregon M.J., 2014; Sebo Z.L., Rodeheffer M.S., 2019).

During maturation, adipocytes undergo complex remodeling that includes hypertrophy (size increase) alongside active lipid biosynthesis. With aging or shifts in external conditions, adipocytes can move between functional states, adjusting both structure and behavior, which ultimately influence overall adipose tissue health.

This multistage maturation pathway underlies adipose tissue's adaptability and its role in metabolism. Understanding the steps and regulatory mechanisms of adipocyte formation is therefore essential for studying metabolic disease and for developing effective interventions (Song T., Kuang S., 2019).

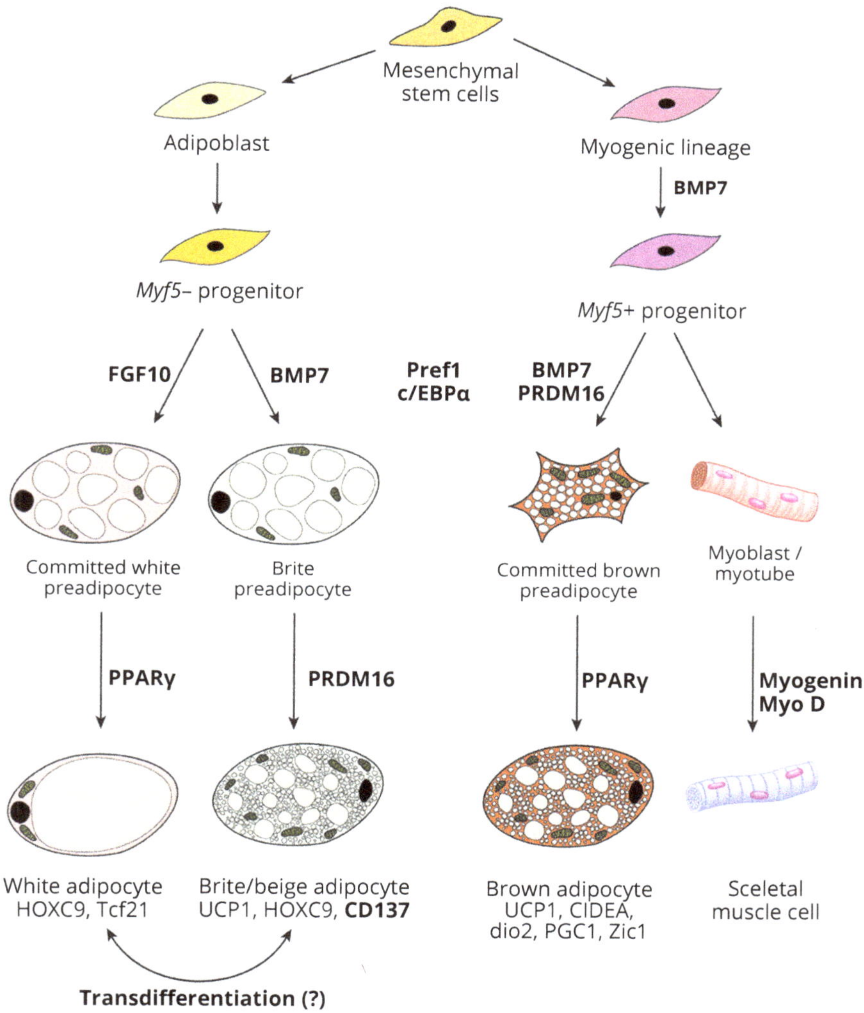

Fig. I-1-2. Developmental pathways of different adipocyte types and key molecular markers involved in adipogenic differentiation (adapted from Obregon M.J., 2014; CC BY)

Abbreviations: BMP7 — bone morphogenetic protein 7 (osteogenic protein-7); c/EBPα — CCAAT enhancer-binding protein alpha; CD137 — membrane protein, a receptor from the tumor necrosis factor receptor superfamily; CIDEA — cell death activator CIDE-A; dio2 — type 2 deiodinase; HOXC9 — homeobox gene C9; FGF10 — fibroblast growth factor 10; PGC1 — peroxisome proliferator-activated receptor coactivator 1; PPARγ — peroxisome proliferator-activated receptor gamma; PRDM16 — transcription factor 16 containing zinc finger-type domains; Pref1 — preadipocyte factor 1; Tcf21 — transcription factor 21 (epicardin); UCP1 — uncoupling protein 1 (thermogenin); Zic1 — transcription factor 1 from the ZIC family (cerebellar zinc finger proteins)

Table I-1-1. Variety of adipocyte types (adapted from He N. et al., 2023; CC BY)

Phenotype	WHITE	BROWN	BEIGE	PINK	YELLOW
	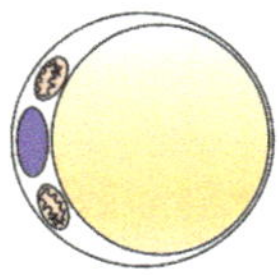	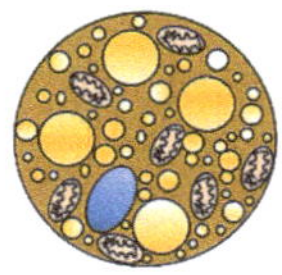	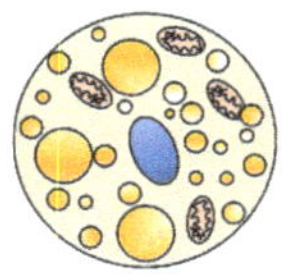	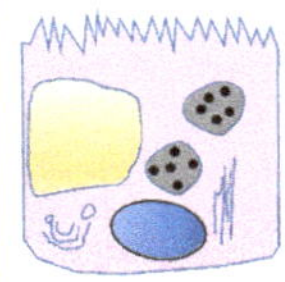	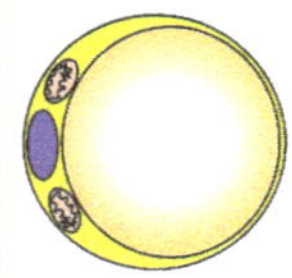
Location	Widely distributed in subcutaneous tissue and around visceral organs	Predominantly in the interscapular region	In adults, located subcutaneously near the spine and collarbone	Develops in breast tissue during pregnancy (conversion from white adipocytes)	Located in the bone marrow cavity
Key feature	• One large lipid droplet occupying most of the cell volume • Low mitochondrial density	• Numerous small lipid droplets • High mitochondrial content	• Numerous small lipid droplets • High mitochondrial content	• One medium-sized lipid droplet • Low mitochondrial density	• One large lipid droplet occupying most of the cell volume • Low mitochondrial density
Primary functions	• Energy storage • Endocrine function (energy balance, reproduction, carbohydrate and lipid metabolism, immune function, etc.) • Mechanical and thermal protection	• Thermogenesis • Regulation of carbohydrate and lipid metabolism (lipid and glucose utilization) • Endocrine function	• Thermogenesis or energy storage • Regulation of carbohydrate and lipid metabolism (lipid and glucose utilization) • Endocrine function	• Reproductive support: energy supply to breast tissue; synthesis and secretion of breast milk	• Bone remodeling • Regulation of hematopoiesis • Endocrine function (e.g., a source of adiponectin during energy deficiency)

1.2.2. Types of adipocytes

Five adipocyte types have been described, differing in structure and function (**Table I-1-1**) (Frigolet M.E., Gutiérrez-Aguilar R., 2020; Zinngrebe J. et al., 2020; He N. et al., 2023).

White adipocytes

White adipocytes are the most common fat cell type. They contain a single large lipid droplet that can occupy up to 90% of the cell volume. The nucleus, along with a small number of mitochondria and other organelles, is displaced toward the cell periphery. The main lipid droplet consists primarily of triglycerides, with smaller amounts of cholesterol esters. Because this droplet appears pale under light microscopy, the cell often looks almost white.

The spherical shape of the white adipocyte allows it to occupy a large volume within a relatively limited space, supporting its primary role — efficient energy storage. White adipocytes also contribute to endocrine regulation by producing leptin*, a hormone involved in energy balance, neuroendocrine signaling, and metabolic regulation. Adipose tissue dominated by white adipocytes also provides thermal insulation and mechanical cushioning for organs.

Brown adipocytes

Brown adipocytes contain many small lipid droplets and abundant mitochondria. They are typically polygonal and about half the size of white adipocytes. The round nucleus is usually positioned centrally. Their numerous large mitochondria contain dense lamellar cristae, consistent with high metabolic activity. The brown coloration reflects high mitochondrial cytochrome content.

Small clusters of brown adipocytes are mainly found in the upper thorax. Their primary function is thermogenesis — heat production through fat oxidation rather than muscle activity. This is especially important for newborns, who have limited thermoregulatory capacity because of low muscle activity, and for animals living in cold environments. Adults retain smaller brown fat reserves, most commonly in the neck and shoulder regions.

Beige adipocytes

Beige adipocytes are intermediate between white and brown adipocytes. Their appearance depends on the functional state. At rest, they resemble white adipocytes (pale cells with a single dominant lipid droplet). When activated, they take on a brown-like appearance, with abundant mitochondria and multiple lipid droplets. Beige adipocytes are concentrated within SAT.

Pink adipocytes

Pink adipocytes are specialized fat cells that develop in breast tissue during pregnancy and lactation. Their pink hue reflects the increased

---

* Leptin is used as a clinical and laboratory marker of risk for type 2 diabetes and coronary heart disease, and it is also used in the diagnosis of obesity and secondary amenorrhea.

vascularity of the mammary gland during this period. Pink adipocytes contribute to milk synthesis and secretion and also produce adipokines (hormone-like signaling molecules released by adipose tissue). Importantly, this phenotype is reversible: after lactation ends, pink adipocytes revert to white adipocytes, restoring adipose content within the mammary gland.

Yellow adipocytes

Yellow adipocytes are found in bone marrow and resemble white adipocytes in overall structure, with one large lipid droplet. In yellow adipocytes, triglycerides contain a higher proportion of saturated fatty acids, and the yellow coloration is attributed to a high carotenoid concentration within the lipid droplets. Compared with subcutaneous adipocytes, yellow adipocytes show minimal lipolytic response to adrenergic stimulation, which helps explain why their numbers change little during caloric restriction. They also have relatively high glucose uptake capacity compared with white adipocytes, but are resistant to insulin-stimulated glucose uptake. Yellow adipocytes additionally participate in the regulation of hematopoiesis and bone formation.

1.2.3. Distribution of adipocytes

In adults, adipose tissue is composed primarily of white adipocytes, which are optimized for long-term energy storage and gradual release. These cells contain relatively few mitochondria, and lipids are stored in a single large droplet, further slowing their mobilization. In contrast, brown adipocytes — abundant in newborns and critical for temperature maintenance — contain many mitochondria and minor lipid inclusions.

Thermogenic brown adipose tissue has a dense capillary network (up to 5 per cell) and rich sympathetic innervation. Its morphology changes with age. In infants and across the first decade of life, adipocytes with multiple lipid droplets predominate; in adults, brown adipose tissue becomes more heterogeneous, with cells containing one or several droplets, often with higher overall lipid content.

A key marker of thermogenic adipocytes is thermogenin (UCP1). This protein is located in the inner mitochondrial membrane and is required for non-shivering thermogenesis. In infants, it plays a vital role in limiting heat loss, which would otherwise be substantial due to the high surface area-to-volume ratio. Beige adipocytes also express UCP1, but at lower levels. UCP1 is not detected in white adipocytes (Nie T. et al., 2023).

Fat cells are highly plastic and can undergo transdifferentiation, shifting between states (**Fig. I-1-3**). This adaptive capacity is especially relevant when addressing obesity and metabolic disease. Converting white adipose tissue into beige or brown phenotypes increases energy expenditure and supports metabolic improvement (Sakers A. et al., 2022; Peng Y. et al., 2024).

Browning is most pronounced in inguinal SAT, while it is less efficient in visceral adipose tissue. This shift is linked to increased mitochondrial activity and higher heat production through thermogenesis. Physical activity (for example, high-intensity interval training), cold exposure, and prolonged fasting can promote browning.

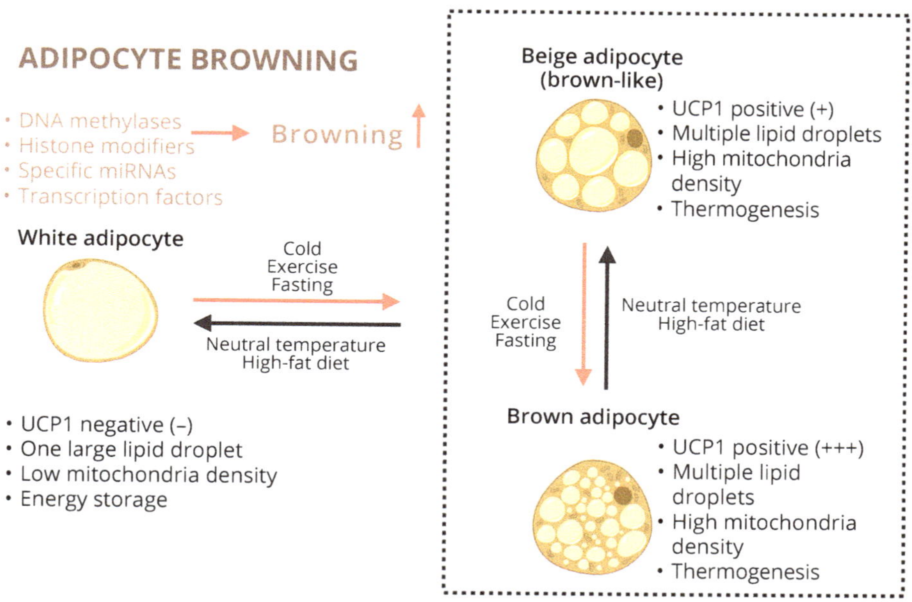

Fig. I-1-3. Three types of adipocyte interactions and browning. Image created with BioRender.com (adapted from Peng Y. et al., 2024; CC BY)

Beige cells represent an intermediate stage and, over time, may progress toward a brown like phenotype, which is associated with activation of thermogenic function.

In some situations, transdifferentiation can also proceed in the opposite direction: brown and beige adipocytes may acquire white adipocyte features, favoring energy storage over heat production. This process, known as whitening, may contribute to challenges in weight control (see Part II, section 3.1). From a practical standpoint, understanding how to maintain and enhance thermogenic activity in brown and beige adipose tissue is essential for supporting metabolic regulation and body weight management (Mo Y.Y. et al., 2024).

1.3. Fat metabolism

1.3.1. Triglycerides: the primary component of fat

Fats are organic compounds that are esters formed when carboxylic acids (fatty acids) are esterified with the trihydric alcohol glycerol to form triglycerides (**Fig. I-1-4**). The fatty acid composition of a triglyceride determines the physical properties of the fat at room temperature: the more unsaturated the fatty acids, the higher the melting point, resulting in a more liquid fat.

In everyday language, products containing fats are described as "oil", "butter", or "fat". A fat that is liquid at room temperature is typically called an "oil", while a solid fat is commonly described as "butter" or "fat". Most vegetable oils (such as sunflower, olive, and soybean)

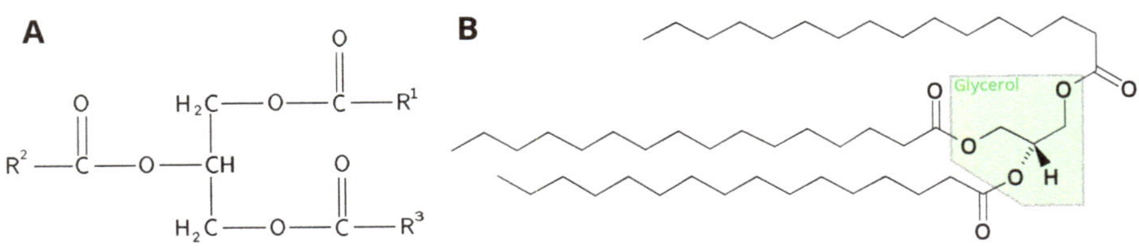

Fig. I-1-4. Triglycerides: A — overall structure of the molecule (R^1, R^2, and R^3 — fatty acids); B — example: tripalmitin, consisting of a glycerol backbone (shown in green) esterified to three identical palmitic acid chains (Wikipedia)

are liquid, but solid vegetable butters also exist, including palm, coconut, and cocoa. Most animal fats are solid and remain firm at room temperature, with some exceptions, such as fish oil.

1.3.2. Lipogenesis and lipolysis: the two sides of fat metabolism

Triglycerides are the body's universal energy reserve: excess intake of essential nutrients (lipids, carbohydrates, and proteins) can be converted into triglycerides and stored in adipocytes when caloric intake exceeds energy needs.

Lipogenesis, the synthesis of lipids in the body, is one of the most critical mechanisms governing energy balance. A primary substrate for fat synthesis is acetyl coenzyme A (acetyl CoA), generated during mitochondrial carbohydrate processing. In hepatocytes, acetyl-CoA is converted through sequential reactions into fatty acids, which then combine with proteins to form low-density lipoproteins (LDL). LDL enter the bloodstream and reach adipose tissue, where lipids are ultimately stored as triglycerides.

When nutrient availability is limited, triglycerides are broken down into free fatty acids (FFA) and glycerol — this process is known as **lipolysis**. Fatty acids are released from adipocytes into the bloodstream and circulate in association with lipoprotein particles (chylomicrons). In peripheral tissues, specific enzymes liberate fatty acids from these particles, enabling cellular uptake and metabolism.

Unused fatty acids bind to albumin. Oxidation ("burning") of fatty acids — their breakdown into carbon dioxide and water with energy release — occurs in mitochondria.

Certain hormones, including insulin, estrogen, and prolactin, promote lipid accumulation (lipogenesis) in adipocytes. Lipid breakdown (lipolysis) is enhanced by testosterone, epinephrine, norepinephrine, glucagon, human growth hormone (HGH), and cortisol.

When fat accumulates in large amounts, white adipocytes markedly increase in volume and adipose tissue undergoes **hypertrophy**. Once their capacity for expansion is exhausted, adipose tissue-derived stem cells (ADSCs) are activated, and new adipocytes form — adipose tissue **hyperplasia** develops (Saponaro C. et al., 2015).

1.4. Other cells of adipose tissue

In addition to adipocytes, adipose tissue contains multiple other cell populations (Esteve Ràfols M., 2014). These include mature, specialized cells as well as stem and low-differentiated cells. Together, they confer adipose tissue with strong regenerative potential and help explain why it is increasingly used in regenerative medicine.

A primary focus is the so-called **stromal vascular fraction (SVF)** — a heterogeneous cell mixture obtained from lipoaspirate by separating mature adipocytes from the remaining cellular components (**Fig. I-1-5**).

Key SVF cellular components include:

- **Adipose-derived stem cells (ADSCs):** Multipotent cells capable of differentiating into multiple tissue types, including bone, cartilage, muscle, and fat. ADSCs are a core SVF component and a major contributor to its regenerative potential.
- **Preadipocytes:** Adipocyte precursor cells that can differentiate into mature adipocytes.
- **Endothelial cells:** Mature endothelial cells line the inner surface of blood vessels, while endothelial progenitor cells support new vessel formation during angiogenesis.
- **Immune cells:** Macrophages, T-lymphocytes, and other immune cells play central roles in inflammation and immune regulation.
- **Pericytes:** Cells located on the outer surface of capillaries. Their processes can encircle a microvessel or extend longitudinally. Pericytes are essential for stabilizing microvessels and regulating vascular permeability.
- **Fibroblasts:** Cells that produce extracellular matrix and provide structural support during tissue repair and regeneration.

Because of these regenerative properties, SVF has a wide range of potential medical applications that are actively being studied and gradually entering clinical practice (Bora P., Majumdar A.S., 2017; Kostecka A. et al., 2024). SVF has been investigated for cartilage regeneration in osteoarthritis and other joint disorders, as well as for bone repair in fractures and other osseous defects. SVF also promotes

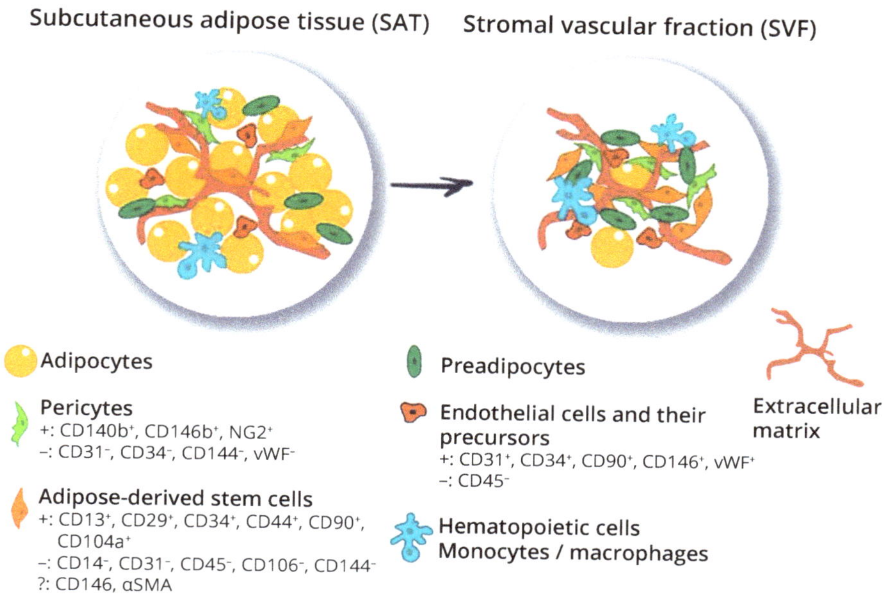

Fig. I-1-5. Cellular composition of SAT and SVF

angiogenesis and may support perfusion in conditions such as coronary heart disease, obliterative atherosclerosis, and other vascular disorders. In addition, SVF-driven immune modulation may be relevant for autoimmune diseases such as rheumatoid arthritis and multiple sclerosis.

Evidence supporting dermatologic applications of SVF is also growing (Jafarzadeh A. et al., 2024). SVF may support burn repair (Fakiha K., 2022), promote healing of chronic wounds such as diabetic ulcers (Moon K.C. et al., 2019), improve skin status in systemic scleroderma (Guillaume-Jugnot P. et al., 2016), and support scar management (Mbiine R. et al., 2022). In trichology, SVF may improve graft take of transplanted hair follicles, slow hair loss, and enhance hair growth and quality (Mantovani G.P. et al., 2023). In aesthetic medicine, SVF is used to support overall skin quality and rejuvenation (Surowiecka A., Strużyna J., 2022).

SVF is administered by injection into the affected area.

1.5. Adipose tissue as an endocrine organ

Adipose tissue was initially viewed as an inert "storage" organ with basic functions of nutrient accumulation and release. It later became clear that adipose cells synthesize and secrete multiple hormones and regulatory mediators (Kershaw E.E., Flier J.S., 2004). These include leptin, interleukin-6 (IL-6), tumor necrosis factor alpha (TNF-α), transforming growth factor beta (TGF-β), angiotensin, vascular endothelial growth factor (VEGF), fibroblast growth factor (FGF), and many others (Lafontan M., 2014). They act systemically and participate in a wide range of physiologic and pathologic processes.

In addition, during premenopause and menopause, adipose tissue can contribute to the production of female sex hormones, which may partially offset adverse effects associated with reproductive decline (Ou M.Y. et al., 2022). In this way, adipose tissue can influence energy balance, appetite regulation, and multiple metabolic pathways.

1.6. Aging of adipose tissue

Aging of adipose tissue is a complex, multifactorial process and is directly relevant when discussing strategies that support healthy aging and reduce the risk of age-associated diseases.

One key change is structural remodeling with functional decline: in older individuals, adipose tissue becomes more fibrotic, the number of metabolically active adipocytes decreases, and the connective tissue component increases. This is associated with immune cell migration (including macrophages and T lymphocytes) and the development of low-grade chronic inflammation known as inflammaging. Chronic adipose-tissue inflammation is linked to multiple long-term conditions and age-related changes, including shifts in skin status and reduced thermoregulation.

At the same time, adipocytes become less effective at storing energy and secreting adipokines, which negatively affects metabolism, including glucose and lipid handling.

Fat distribution also shifts with age: subcutaneous fat tends to decline, while internal depots, especially visceral fat, increase (**Fig. I-1-6**).

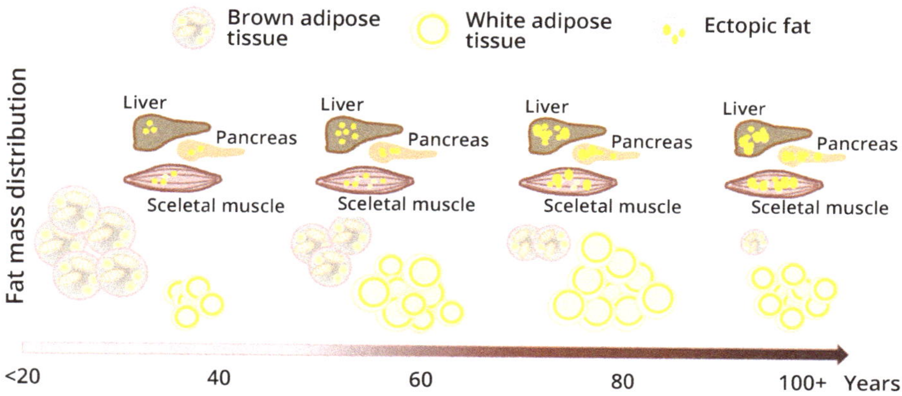

Fig. I-1-6. Age-related remodeling of fat mass. From birth through older age, both the amount and distribution of fat change: white adipose tissue increases in adipocyte number and size, while brown adipose tissue declines. In parallel, fat can accumulate in non-typical locations (ectopic fat), including the liver, skeletal muscle, and pancreas. Ectopic fat may disrupt cellular processes, impair organ function, and be associated with insulin resistance (adapted from Conte M. et al., 2019; CC BY)

This redistribution is associated with poorer metabolic health and a higher risk of cardiovascular disease and metabolic syndrome (Conte M. et al., 2019).

Collectively, these processes contribute to metabolic disturbances, including insulin resistance, type 2 diabetes, and dyslipidemia.

1.7. Aesthetic problems related and not related to SAT

A skincare professional cannot meaningfully target visceral fat or the deep subcutaneous fat layer — specifically, the depots that undergo hypertrophy in obesity — although some modern device-based interventions do offer options that may influence these compartments.

By contrast, many aesthetic concerns are linked to the subcutaneous fat layer, which can respond more predictably to aesthetic interventions. These concerns include contour irregularities in the abdomen and thighs (often described as cellulite) and localized adipose accumulation in the chin, jawline, neck, and shoulders. These zones are typical targets of sculpting procedures.

It is also worth noting that patient concerns do not always fall within the scope of body-contouring practice. The presenting issue may involve neither excess adipose tissue nor cellulite.

For example, **abdominal prominence** may be associated with:

- Muscle imbalance in the lower back and pelvic region, with some muscle groups overactive and others weakened (lower crossed syndrome)
- Weakness of the anterior abdominal-wall musculature
- Diastasis of the *rectus abdominis*, with separation of the muscle bellies along the linea alba due to weakening and stretching (commonly postpartum)
- Lumbar spine curvature abnormalities, including excessive lordosis or reduced lordosis (flattening)
- Postural disorders affecting balance control, gait, and posture
- Visceral dysfunction accompanied by mesenteric edema (intra-abdominal lymphostasis)

"Dimples" in the buttocks may reflect differences in tone across the gluteal group — specifically, hypotonia of the gluteus maximus combined with hypertonia of the gluteus medius and minimus.

Surface irregularities on the outer thigh are not always a sign of SAT hypertrophy; they may also result from dysfunction of the deep fascia of the thigh (*fascia lata*).

When these patterns are identified, the preferred strategy typically includes therapeutic massage, orthopedic care, physical therapy, and exercise therapy.

Chapter 2
Cellulite

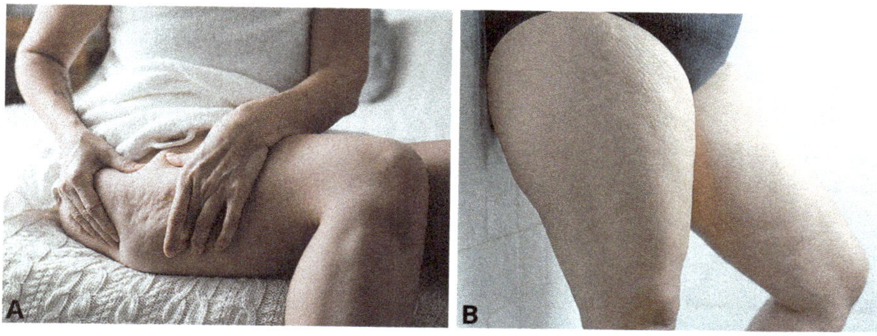

Fig. I-2-1. Cellulite at early (A) and late (B) stages (Photo: Freepik)

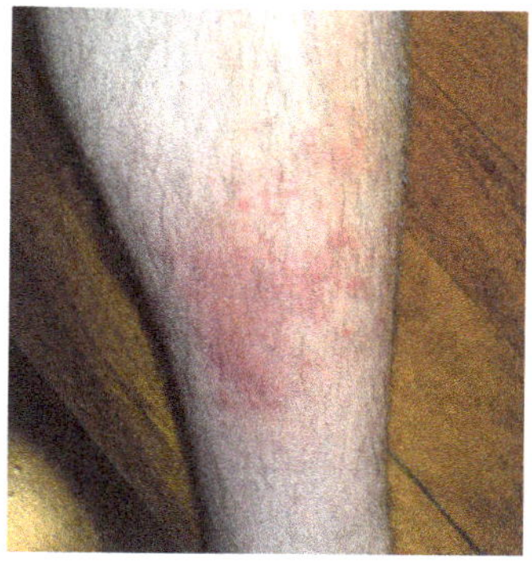

Fig. I-2-2. Infection-related cellulitis (Photo: RafaelLopez / Wikipedia)

Structural changes in the SAT can lead to the aesthetic concern commonly called "orange peel" texture (**cellulite**). It is characterized by an uneven surface and palpable lumpiness that, in early stages, may be visible only when the skin is pinched (**Fig. I-2-1A**) and, in later stages, persists even at rest (**Fig. I 2-1B**). Cellulite most often affects the thighs and buttocks and is not considered a disease. To avoid confusion with **cellulitis** (a suppurative inflammation, or phlegmon, of the SAT) (**Fig. I-2-2**), aesthetic cellulite is sometimes referred to as gynoid lipodystrophy. However, the term "cellulite" is firmly established in cosmetic dermatology and aesthetic medicine; in this book, we will use it in its usual sense as understood by skincare professionals.

Related structural shifts may also contribute to localized fat pockets in the chin, jawline, neck, and shoulder regions. These deposits, together with areas of cellulite, can be targets for aesthetic procedures, which we will discuss in Part II.

2.1. Causes of cellulite

Cellulite is predominantly a female concern. Although the literature does not provide reliable epidemiologic prevalence data, published estimates suggest that cellulite is present in 80–90% of postpubertal women (Friedmann D.P. et al., 2017; Gabriel A. et al., 2023). In men, cellulite is uncommon, even with obesity and reduced tissue tone, but it can occur in conditions associated with androgen deficiency or in patients receiving estrogen therapy.

A key reason is the sex-specific architecture of SAT. In men, the fibrous septa that partition adipose tissue into lobules tend to run at an angle toward the skin surface. In women, these septa are oriented more perpendicular to the surface. In addition, male lobules are smaller, so skin texture tends to change less even as adipocytes enlarge. In women, dimpling and lumpiness are more likely to develop (**Fig. I-2-3**).

The root cause of cellulite remains debated. One view holds that cellulite begins with localized hypertrophy of adipocytes under the influence of female sex hormones, which is why it tends to develop in reproductively significant regions (abdomen, thighs, buttocks). In this framework, its severity may fluctuate with the menstrual cycle and is influenced by pregnancy and menopause.

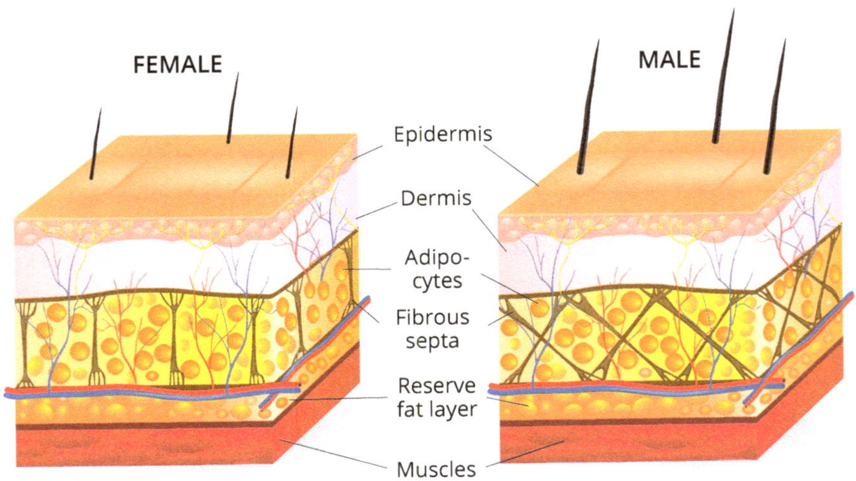

Fig. I-2-3. Female-male differences in SAT structure (Image: Designua/ Shutterstock)

Another view places connective-tissue remodeling at the center of the process, with disrupted microcirculation as the trigger and other changes developing secondarily.

Some authors propose that cellulite begins with disturbances in the microcirculation of blood and lymph within the SAT. In this model, edema and hypoxia promote capillary neoformation, fibrosis, and thickening of connective tissue septa (Omi T. et al., 2013). Other authors dispute this interpretation, noting that evidence is insufficient to conclude that vascular and lymphatic impairment is the primary driver of cellulite (Friedmann D.P. et al., 2017).

Another hypothesis focuses on the endocrine and signaling activity of adipocytes (Li J. et al., 2014). Specific pro-inflammatory cytokines may promote septal fibrosis within SAT. A decrease in adiponectin expression — a hormone known for anti-inflammatory, antifibrotic, and vasodilatory effects — has also been discussed as a contributor to cellulite pathogenesis in women with associated conditions (Emanuele E. et al., 2011). In addition, during premenopause and menopause, adipose tissue can contribute to the production of female sex hormones, which may partially buffer adverse effects associated with reproductive decline.

Adipose tissue plays a central role in regulating energy balance, appetite, and the metabolism of many substances. Under typical conditions, without adipocyte hypertrophy and degenerative changes in connective tissue and vessels, adipocyte-released mediators enter the bloodstream and reach target organs without major impediment. When circulation is compromised, however, fluid can accumulate around adipocytes, increasing local concentrations of cytokines and hormones. Instead of dispersing systemically, these mediators may remain within adipose tissue and act locally. In this context, female sex hormones can promote lipogenesis and alter lymphatic vessel tone, contributing to lymphatic stasis, while TNF-α can promote inflammation.

It is also important to remember that adipose tissue serves as a reservoir not only for nutrients, but also for endotoxins and metabolic byproducts that are ordinarily cleared via lymphatic flow. When microcirculation is impaired, these substances, along with lipids, can accumulate within adipocytes, further aggravating microcirculatory disturbances and contributing to metabolic imbalance in adipose tissue (**Fig. I-2-4**).

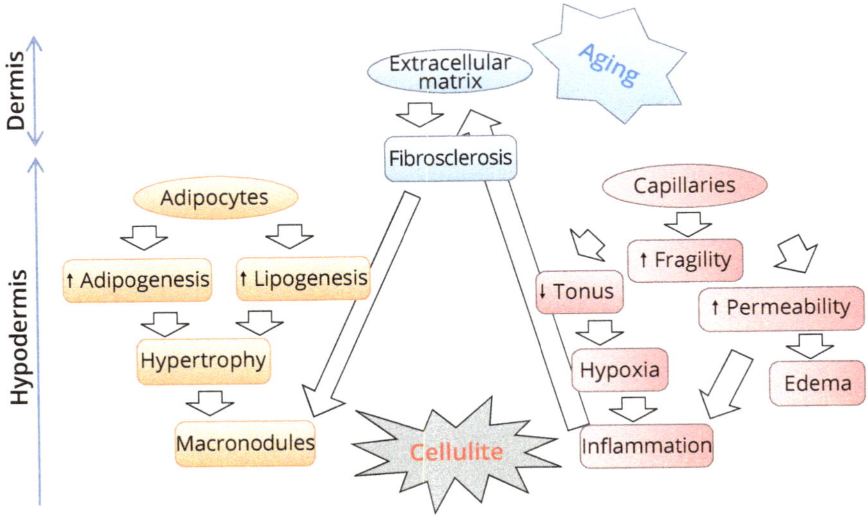

Fig. I-2-4. Core mechanisms associated with cellulite. The exact cause of cellulite remains a matter of debate. Still, most scientists agree that decreased microcirculation, interstitial fluid infiltration (edema), localized adipocyte hypertrophy, oxidative stress, persistent low-grade inflammation, and changes in the extracellular matrix contribute to its development. Cellulite and skin aging may influence each other (adapted from Dupont E. et al., 2014; CC BY)

2.2. Stages and symptoms

Cellulite begins with localized hypertrophy of fat lobules or, more precisely, with local lipodystrophy — an imbalance between lipogenesis (fat synthesis) and lipolysis (fat breakdown) within adipocytes. Unlike obesity, where fat accumulation is more uniform, cellulite involves uneven deposition across discrete adipocyte clusters.

Four stages are typically described.

Stage 1

- Skin changes not visibly apparent; findings detectable only on histology
- Reduced capillary density with impaired perfusion of adipose tissue

- Occasional pallor and mild puffiness
- Damage to the collagen–elastin network
- Adipocyte enlargement by 2–3 times with clustering into "islands" and reduced tissue uniformity
- Early extracellular fluid accumulation

Stage 2

- Ongoing connective tissue disruption with continued vessel loss
- Further adipocyte enlargement with larger "islands" and peripheral displacement of vessels
- Progressive interstitial fluid accumulation
- Normal appearing skin at rest, with "orange peel" texture on pinching

Stage 3

- Continuation of stage 2 changes
- Connective tissue sheath formation around adipocyte "islands"
- Dermal thinning with protrusion of fat nodules into the dermis
- Visible "orange peel" texture without pinching

Stage 4

- Dense, painful nodules in adipose tissue with compression of nerve endings and protrusion into the dermis
- Cold skin sensation with a bluish hue
- Marked surface irregularities and bumpiness

Some authors also describe a fifth stage marked by pronounced edema and inflammatory changes with pain, and by the presence of cellulite on the hands. At the same time, the first three stages are typically approached as aesthetic concerns, while the fourth and fifth stages are considered pathological.

Chapter 3
Obesity: What to expect in the skin?

Obesity is a heterogeneous group of inherited and acquired diseases characterized by excessive accumulation of adipose tissue (**Table I-3-1**). The World Health Organization defines obesity as the accumulation of abnormal or excessive fat deposits that may be detrimental to health.

Table I-3-1. Classification of obesity (Peterkova V.A., Vasyukova O.V., 2015)

OBESITY TYPE	CAUSE
By etiology	
Simple (exogenous-constitutional, idiopathic)	Excess calorie intake combined with hypodynamia and hereditary predisposition
Hypothalamic	Hypothalamic and brainstem tumors and their treatment; radiation therapy for brain tumors and hemoblastosis; cranial trauma or stroke
Obesity in neuroendocrine diseases	Hypercorticism, hypothyroidism, etc.
Iatrogenic obesity	Prolonged use of glucocorticoids, antidepressants, and some other drugs
Monogenic obesity	Mutations in genes encoding leptin, leptin receptor, melanocortin receptors 3 and 4, proopiomelanocortin, proconvertase type 1, and neurotrophic factor receptor (tropomyosin related kinase B)
Syndromal obesity	Chromosomal and other genetic syndromes — Prader Willi, fragile X chromosome, Alström, Cohen, Down, pseudohypoparathyroidism, etc.

Continued on p. 35

Beginning of the Table I-3-1 on p. 34

OBESITY TYPE	CAUSE
By complications and comorbid conditions	
Carbohydrate metabolism disorders	Diabetes mellitus type 2
Non-alcoholic fatty liver disease	Gallstone disease
Dyslipidemia	Hyperandrogenism syndrome
Arterial hypertension	Musculoskeletal disorders
Delayed sexual development	Gynecomastia
Accelerated sexual development	Apnea syndrome
By degree of obesity (by % above "ideal" body weight)	
I degree	15–24.9%
II degree	25–49.9%
III degree	50–99.9%
Morbid	> 100%

The **body mass index (BMI)**, which is calculated as the ratio of weight (kg) to body length squared, expressed in meters, is a universal criterion for weight assessment:

$$BMI = weight\ (kg) / height^2\ (m).$$

- Underweight: BMI < 19 (women) and < 20 (men)
- Normal weight: BMI 19–20 (women) and 20–25 (men)
- Slightly overweight: BMI 24–30 (women) and 25–30 (men)
- Tendency to obesity: BMI 30–40
- Obesity: BMI ≥ 30

Overweight is a problem whose incidence has risen rapidly over the past few decades. While its aesthetic implications are interpreted differently today (with the body positive movement challenging established stereotypes), obesity carries substantial health risks. Along with excess weight, multiple disorders can affect virtually all organs and systems, including the skin.

Skincare products cannot meaningfully reduce fat volume in patients with obesity, but they can improve overall skin status. This matters because people with obesity often present with multiple skin concerns affecting both small and extensive areas, and some lesions may signal severe underlying disease. For providers working in body contouring, understanding the mechanisms and clinical patterns of obesity associated skin disorders is therefore essential.

3.1. Skin pathophysiology in obesity

Excessive expansion of SAT in obesity is associated with impaired microcirculation and reduced trophic support of the skin. All skin layers may be affected, including the epidermis, which plays a central role in barrier function. The *stratum corneum* retains water less effectively, contributing to reduced hydration and dryness. Barrier integrity may be further compromised by increased activity of sebaceous and sweat glands and by changes in immune status. The skin of patients with obesity often shows higher irritability and greater susceptibility to infection (Hirt P.A. et al., 2019; Rosen J. et al., 2019; Geeta Sai G. et al., 2024; Zaccaron R.P. et al., 2024).

3.1.1. Skin barrier

Altered barrier function has been linked to obesity. **Xerosis** is commonly reported in morbid obesity and is associated with reduced hydration of the *stratum corneum* (Guida B. et al., 2010).

An important marker of barrier function is transepidermal water loss (TEWL). Studies examining TEWL in obesity have produced inconsistent findings. For example, de Farias Pires T. et al. (2016) reported increased TEWL and attributed it to heightened sweating. In contrast, Guida B. et al. (2010) reported decreased TEWL, linking it to increased sebum production and formation of a thicker occlusive film on the skin surface.

Despite elevated sebum levels, the *stratum corneum* may remain dehydrated. This has been attributed to structural changes driven by adipokines. Adipokines promote keratinocyte proliferation, accelerating epidermal cell turnover and preventing normal maturation of the *stratum corneum*. As a result, barrier structures form incompletely, permeability increases, and adequate water retention is not achieved.

3.1.2. Sebaceous glands

Sebum secretion is stimulated by androgens, insulin, human growth hormone (HGH), and insulin-like growth factors, which are often elevated in obesity. As a result, sebum production increases, along with the risk of acne.

3.1.3. Sweat glands

People with obesity often experience increased sweating, supported by both abundant skin folds and a thick SAT layer. Constant friction within folds, together with a moist environment, promotes inflammation. **Intertrigo** develops in areas of maceration and presents as erythematous plaques within folds, followed by secondary infection of fungal or bacterial origin (**Fig. I-3-1**) (Pera F. et al., 2025).

Intertrigo, diabetes, and obesity also facilitate bacterial contamination and may contribute to another pathologic skin condition, bromhidrosis. **Bromhidrosis** results from bacterial and fungal breakdown of sweat, leading to a strong, unpleasant body odor.

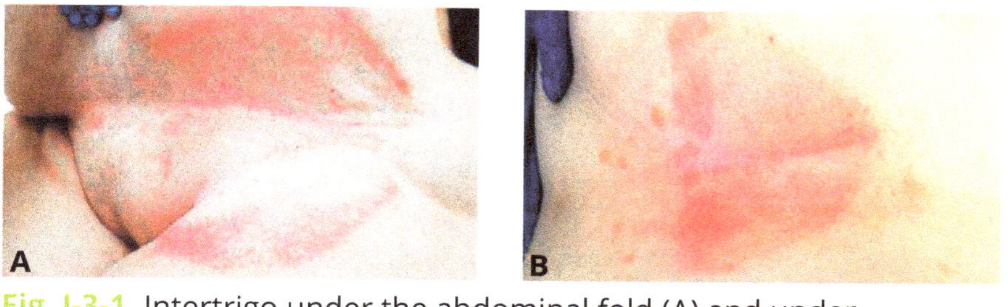

Fig. I-3-1. Intertrigo under the abdominal fold (A) and under the breast (B) in a patient with obesity (adapted from Pera F. et al., 2025; CC BY)

3.1.4. Collagen and wound healing

In animal models, fibroblasts from obese subjects show reduced synthetic activity. Collagen deficiency is observed, and collagen production after skin injury is slower and less robust (Li P. et al., 2005). Clinically, this helps explain reduced skin elasticity and tensile strength in obesity, as well as delayed wound healing.

Leptin resistance is another adverse effect associated with obesity. Leptin plays a key role in wound repair and recovery. When the response to leptin is blunted, healing processes become less effective, and patients with obesity may have greater difficulty achieving normal wound closure and tissue restoration (Shipman A.R., Millington G.W., 2011).

3.1.5. Microcirculatory bed

In obesity, microangiopathy refers to damage affecting small vessels within the microcirculation. It can lead to multiple downstream effects, including venous insufficiency, impaired lymphatic flow, congestion, and hypoxia. At rest, skin capillaries may be maximally filled, reducing the reserve capacity of cutaneous blood flow. Venous stasis is further aggravated by valvular failure and increased intra-abdominal pressure (Vivas A. et al., 2016). A common clinical manifestation in this setting is **venous eczema,** characterized by erythema, dryness, scaling, pruritus, and an increased risk of infection. Lymphatic outflow is also compromised, contributing to lymphedema. Widespread edema, protein-rich interstitial fluid accumulation, and reduced perfusion create a background for ulceration and infection.

3.2. Obesity and skin diseases

Beyond the findings listed above, obesity can directly or indirectly contribute to a wide range of skin diseases (**Fig. I-3-2**). By pathogenesis, they can be grouped into infectious, inflammatory, and metabolic categories (Geeta Sai G. et al., 2024).

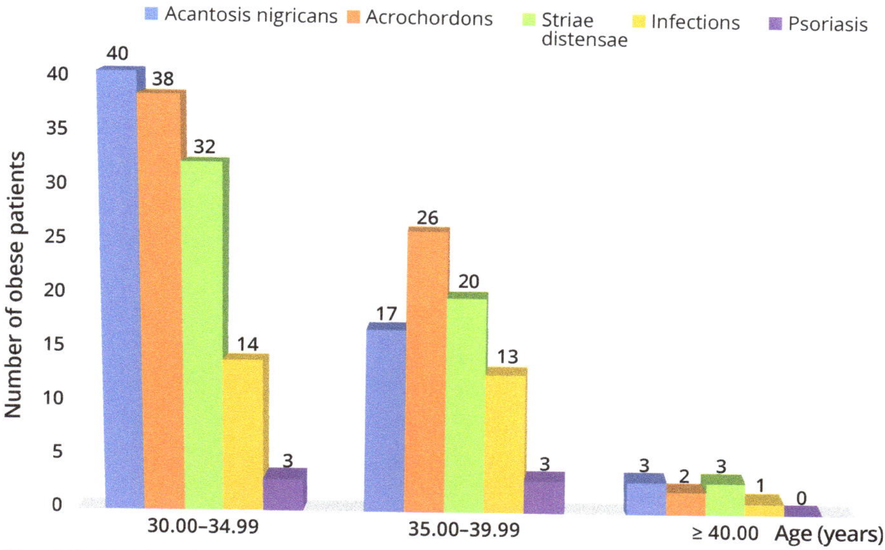

Fig. I-3-2. Distribution (%) of skin manifestations among patients with obesity by BMI (adapted from Geeta Sai G. et al., 2024; CC BY)

Prevalence varies between male and female patients, as shown in a cross-sectional observational study of 100 patients with obesity (**Table I-3-2**) (Geeta Sai G. et al., 2024). Mean age at presentation was 39.3 (±9.9) years. Age distribution included 34% aged 31–40, 30% aged 41–50, 23% aged 19–30, 11% aged 51–60, and 2% over 60. Mean BMI was 34.3 (±2.6). Most participants (63%) had a BMI of 30.00–34.99, 34% had degree II obesity (BMI 35.00–39.99), and 3% had degree III obesity (BMI >40).

Table I-3-2. Relationship between gender and skin pathologies in obese patients (* — statistically significant) (Geeta Sai G. et al., 2024)

SKIN PATHOLOGIES	WOMEN	MEN	*P*-VALUE
Acanthosis nigricans	37 (61.7%)	23 (38.3%)	0.012*
Acrochordon (soft fibroma)	51 (77.3%)	15 (22.7%)	0.054
Striae	40 (72.7%)	15 (27.3%)	0.674
Bacterial infection	1 (25.0%)	3 (75.0%)	0.198
Fungal infection	17 (73.9%)	6 (26.1%)	0.198
Viral infection	1 (100%)	0 (0%)	0.198
Psoriasis	6 (100%)	0 (0%)	0.106

3.2.1. Dermatoses

Purulent hidradenitis (inflammation of the sweat glands) is more common in obese patients. Contributing factors include ductal occlusion, elevated pro-inflammatory cytokines, and skin irritation associated with heavy sweating. Clinical presentation ranges from transient inflammatory nodules to abscesses, fistulas, and subsequent scarring.

Psoriasis severity has been shown to correlate with the degree of obesity (Armstrong A.W. et al., 2012). Clinical observations also suggest that patients with excess weight may require higher medication doses to achieve a therapeutic effect. Weight loss has been reported to have a positive influence on the course of psoriasis (Al Mutairi N., Nour T., 2014).

The association between obesity and **rosacea** is less clear, and published findings are inconsistent. One study reported a positive relationship between increasing BMI and rosacea onset, suggesting that weight gain, particularly earlier in life, may increase susceptibility (Li S. et al., 2017). These data should be interpreted cautiously, and the topic requires further study.

A similar situation applies to **atopic dermatitis**. Several studies, including a meta-analysis, support an association between atopic dermatitis and obesity, with a tendency toward more severe atopy in individuals with excess weight (Zhang A., Silverberg J., 2015).

Premature hair graying is defined as the loss of hair pigmentation before the expected physiologic age threshold, typically before 30 years. One proposed contributor is cortisol. In a study by Papafotiou C. et al. (2017), patients with obesity had elevated salivary cortisol levels, which may play a role in early graying.

3.2.2. Skin infections

Obesity is associated with a higher risk of infectious skin disease and may worsen outcomes, in part because of a pro-inflammatory systemic milieu and reduced T cell-mediated immunity (Huttunen R., Syrjanen J., 2013). Physical inactivity and practical barriers to daily hygiene also contribute. Reported infections and infection-related conditions include candidiasis, folliculitis, furunculosis, erysipelas, erythrasma, necrotizing fasciitis, and, in severe cases, gas gangrene.

Panniculitis (purulent inflammation of the adipose tssue) is more common in patients with obesity and lymphedema, as supported by several systematic reviews (Cannon J. et al., 2018; Taira K.G. et al., 2024).

Excess weight is also associated with **erysipelas** and a higher risk of complications. In studies examining this relationship, obesity was identified as a risk factor for erysipelas and was linked to longer hospital stays. Recurrences were reported even after treatment with a course of benzathine benzylpenicillin (Pitche P. et al., 2015).

Infection of intertriginous dermatitis by *Corynebacterium minutissimum* can result in **erythrasma** — a superficial bacterial infection presenting as reddish brown, finely scaling patches, most often in warm, moist folds such as the axillae, groin, and interdigital spaces. Symptoms may include mild itching. Clinically, it can resemble fungal intertrigo, but diagnosis is straightforward with a Wood's lamp, which shows a coral red fluorescence.

Obesity is a major predisposing factor for **onychomycosis** (Chang S.J. et al., 2008). The reported efficacy of topical antifungal therapy is lower in overweight patients than in those with normal BMI.

Streptococcal elephantiasis (also called elephantiasis nostras verrucosa) is not classic filarial lymphatic elephantiasis. Instead, it is a severe condition driven by chronic bacterial infection (often streptococci) on the background of an already compromised lymphatic system (lymphedema). Clinically, it involves extreme skin thickening with fissuring and verrucous overgrowth, most often affecting the legs or abdomen, with a risk of disability. Management typically includes antibiotics, consistent skin care, and, in select cases, surgical intervention. A vicious cycle can develop: impaired lymphatic drainage enables bacterial overgrowth, inflammation further damages lymphatic function, and swelling and skin changes progressively worsen.

3.2.3. Metabolic disorders

Because obesity often co-exists with metabolic syndrome, patients may present with signs of multiple metabolic disturbances (Chen P.Y. et al., 2019).

Adipose tissue contributes to testosterone production. As adipose volume increases, androgen levels may rise. Obesity is also associated with reduced production of sex hormone-binding globulin, which can further increase serum testosterone (Tchernof A., Després J.P., 2000). **Hyperandrogenism** may be associated with characteristic clinical patterns, including **hirsutism**, **seborrhea**, **acne**, **alopecia**, and **acanthosis nigricans**.

In addition, obesity is common among women with **polycystic ovary syndrome**, a condition characterized by markedly elevated androgen levels.

Tophaceous gout, a disorder of uric acid metabolism, presents primarily with urate deposition in soft tissues. A tophus is a painful, firm nodule that damages surrounding connective tissue and sustains chronic inflammation. The relationship between gout and excess weight is well recognized: obesity is associated with higher uric acid levels, while weight loss can help normalize serum urate levels.

3.3. Common skin manifestations in obesity

Common cutaneous findings in patients with obesity are often linked to metabolic dysregulation and systemic inflammation. Frequent presentations include:

- **Acanthosis nigricans:** Symmetric hyperpigmented patches on the neck, face, flexural surfaces of the extremities, and within skin folds; spot or plaque-like lesions with a verrucous/papillomatous surface; potential complete regression after weight loss
- **Acrochordon ("soft" fibroma)**: Connective tissue growth on a thin stalk; typical sites in friction areas (neck, axillae, groin); possible pruritus
- **Striae:** Erythematous, violaceous, or hypopigmented streaks in regions of pronounced SAT accumulation (abdomen, thighs, lower back)

- **Palmoplantar keratoderma:** Pressure-related damage on the feet with compensatory thickening of the *stratum corneum* on the plantar arch, heel, and hallux
- **Lipodystrophy:** Microcirculatory disturbance in SAT with adipocyte swelling and protrusion of fat lobules, producing "orange peel" skin texture; typical localization on the thighs and buttocks

3.4. Obesity and rare skin conditions

Several rarer skin disorders may be triggered or aggravated by obesity. Although the overall risk in the general population is low, reported cases show direct or indirect links to obesity.

Lipedema is characterized by excessive fat accumulation in the SAT of the lower extremities with progressive enlargement (**Fig. I-3 3**). In severe cases, the trunk and upper body may also be affected. Unlike lymphedema, lipedema involves both legs symmetrically (with sparing of the feet), is typically painless, and occurs exclusively in women. The cause remains unknown, but genetic and hormonal factors are considered likely contributors. Familial clustering is standard, and having an affected relative increases risk. Over time, reduced mobility may develop. Complete recovery is uncommon, but supportive measures can improve function and comfort, including a balanced diet and regular physical activity can help preserve mobility, compression garments to reduce discomfort and support walking, and consistent skincare with moisturizers and emollients

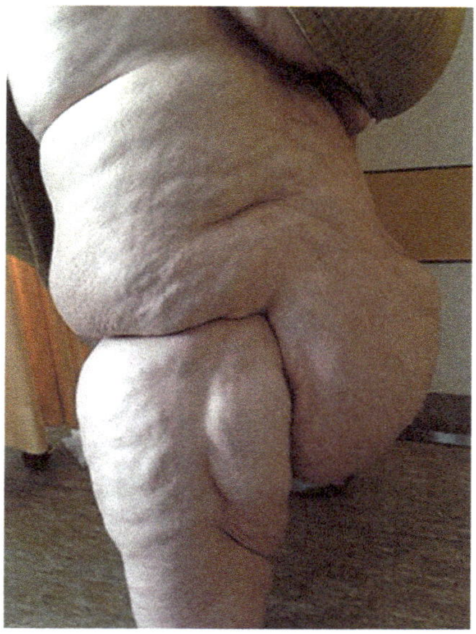

Fig. I-3-3. Advanced lipedema (Photo: Wikimedia)

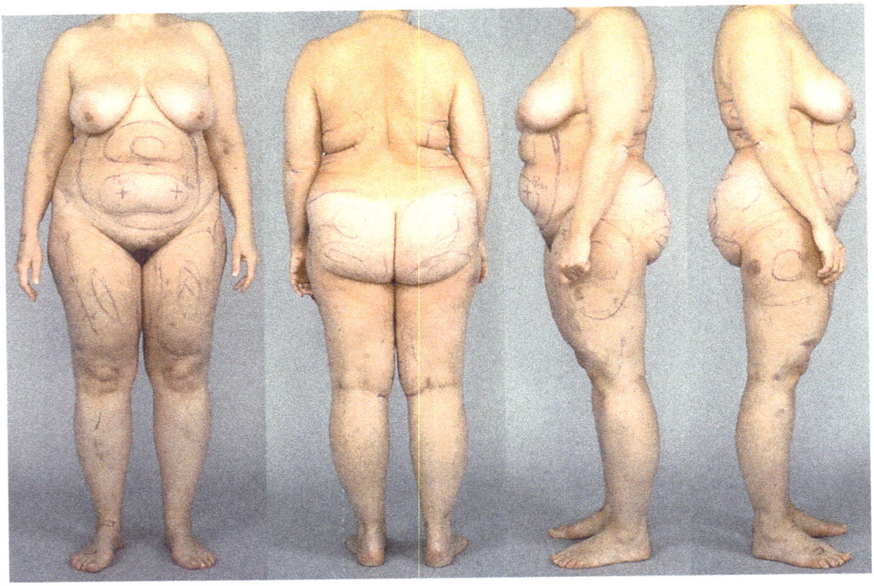

Fig. I-3-4. Patient with Dercum's disease. Type I (generalized, diffuse) form, characterized by painful adipose tissue without clearly demarcated lipomas. The markings shown are preoperative markings before liposuction. Written informed consent was obtained from the patient for publication of this report and accompanying images (adapted from Hansson E. et al., 2012; CC BY)

to reduce xerosis. In advanced cases, liposuction may be considered to reduce fat volume, although it can also injure lymphatic vessels.

Dercum's disease (also called adiposis dolorosa) is a rare, poorly understood autosomal dominant condition characterized by subcutaneous fat deposits in multiple body areas (**Fig. I-3-4**). It has been associated with compression ischemic neuropathy affecting cutaneous branches of peripheral nerves, with clinical features that may include pain, fatigue, and obesity.

Obesity associated lymphedematous mucinosis can resemble pretibial myxedema seen in thyrotoxicosis, although it may not be directly related to thyroid disease. Published reports describe patients with morbid obesity who developed bilateral localized edema of the lower legs that progressed gradually and painlessly, without involving the feet and ankles. Clinical findings included vesicles, translucent papules, or indurated ("woody") plaques on the shins (Ferreli C. et al., 2018). Histology showed characteristic features, including epidermal atrophy with flattening of the dermoepidermal junction, disorganized collagen bundles, increased numbers of capillaries and small vessels with hemosiderin deposition, and mucin accumulation in the papillary dermis and around vessels (Villagrasa-Boli P. et al., 2022).

Overall, excess weight is associated with many skin conditions and can worsen disease course, complicate treatment, and contribute to poorer outcomes. In some patients, topical skincare and standard dermatologic care alone are insufficient. Recognizing the link between obesity and cutaneous pathology early is therefore essential, both to guide management and to support appropriate weight loss counseling.

Part II

Common approaches to subcutaneous adipose tissue remodeling

To initiate the SAT remodeling, two strategies are used:

- **Destructive** — direct disruption of unwanted structures, followed by activation of tissue repair
- **Conservative (physiological restoration)** — targeted support of specific links in physiologic renewal (regeneration) to stimulate change without tissue injury

When choosing a strategy and an approach, it is essential to keep in mind that adipose tissue is a complex system with substantial regenerative capacity. It contains numerous blood vessels and nerve endings. In addition to adipocytes, it includes macrophages, lymphocytes, smooth muscle cells, endothelial cells, and fibroblasts, as well as stem cells capable of differentiating into multiple cell types and serving as a reserve for both SAT and dermal repair (see Part I, section 1.5).

Destruction of adipose tissue affects not only fat cells, but potentially every component of the tissue. For this reason, destructive approaches require caution, especially when the damage is extensive. Large-area injury often promotes inflammation and fibrosis, in part due to vascular disruption. In addition, new adipocytes can form from surviving stem cells and may even outnumber the original population, resulting in SAT hyperplasia.

It is also worth remembering that adipose-tissue functions as an endocrine organ. Aggressive destruction may reduce the body's supply of key mediators and disturb endocrine balance, which further supports a preference for less traumatic options when feasible. Physiologic restoration, a conservative approach to body contouring, accounts for adipocyte hypertrophy and is generally considered safer.

1.1. Scientific substantiation of lipolysis-stimulating strategies

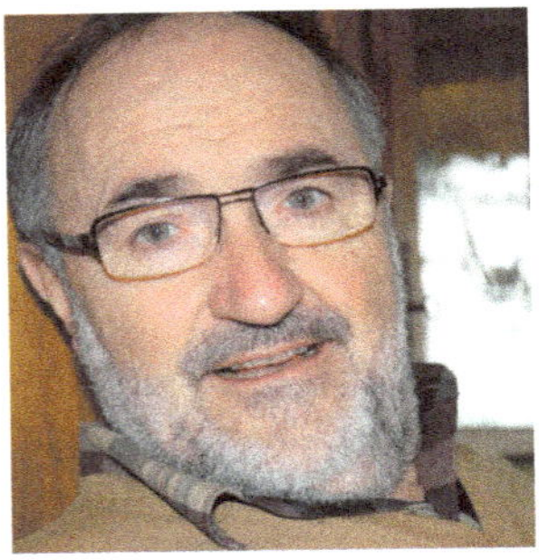

Prof. Max Lafontan

The scientific rationale for this approach is mainly due to the research of Max Lafontan and his colleagues. Prof. Lafontan is one of the most renowned scientists whose career has been closely linked to adipose tissue research for many years. In 1985, he joined the French Institute for Medical Research (Inserm) as Director of Research and was head of Inserm 317 from 1988 to 2003. In 2003, his contributions to the study of adipose-tissue metabolism and obesity were recognized with the Frederick Wasserman Award. Key discoveries made under his leadership include.

- Identification of α2-adrenergic receptors and receptors for neuropeptide Y in adipocytes
- Establishment of molecular mechanisms of interaction between β- and α2-adrenergic receptors in adipocytes of different types
- Study of lysophosphatidic acid synthesis in adipocytes, enabling identification of new substances (e.g., autotaxin, a lysophospholipase involved in lysophosphatidic acid synthesis)
- Discovery of the role of atrial natriuretic peptide in regulating lipolysis and lipid mobilization in humans in 2000, opening a new avenue for research (Lafontan M., 2008; Lafontan M., Langin D., 2009)

Lafontan developed a technique to assess the lipolytic response of adipose tissue to various external stimuli (Monteux C., Lafontan M., 2008). By employing two approaches — microdialysis, a functional tool for evaluating adipose tissue, and DNA microarray analysis, which enables broad gene profiling — he identified significant differences in adipocyte sensitivity among individuals and across different body regions. Notably, the study found the following patterns in the body's response to physical activity:

- Stronger response to physical activity in women with obesity compared with men with obesity (Marques M.A. et al., 2011)
- Detectable exercise-associated lipolysis in adipose tissue of lean individuals, with minimal or absent response in individuals with obesity
- Meaningful reduction of fat deposits with regular exercise in athletes

In untrained individuals with obesity, the lipolytic response of adipose tissue improves gradually after 4 months of 1.5 hours of daily exercise.

A significant advancement in understanding adipose-tissue physiology occurred in 2012 with the discovery of beige adipocytes, fat cells that occupy an intermediate position between brown and white adipocytes. Research on beige cells has shown that they differ fundamentally from both white and brown adipocytes while sharing characteristics of each (Wu J. et al., 2013).

It is important to note that, unlike white adipocytes, brown adipocytes do not store fat; instead, they generate a considerable amount of heat to help maintain body temperature (see Part I, section 1.2). This helps explain why brown fat is prevalent in mammals living in cold climates. It is also present in newborns, comprising about 5% of their tissue, because they require an internal "furnace" for heat generation due to limited muscle activity in the first months of life. Over time, brown fat is gradually replaced by white fat, but some islets persist. Contrary to previous beliefs, brown adipocytes do not entirely lose their function in adults; they were confirmed in adults by 2009, particularly around the neck, shoulders, and upper chest (**Fig. II-1**).

Furthermore, the amount of brown fat in adults increases in cold environments, consistent with its role in thermogenesis. Subsequent studies showed that adult brown fat is fundamentally different from "infant" brown fat: it consists of fat cells formed under the influence of irisin* from precursor cells located within white adipose tissue. These

* Irisin is a hormone released by muscles in response to physical activity. It affects adipose-tissue metabolism (and possibly transdifferentiation), shifting it toward thermogenesis.

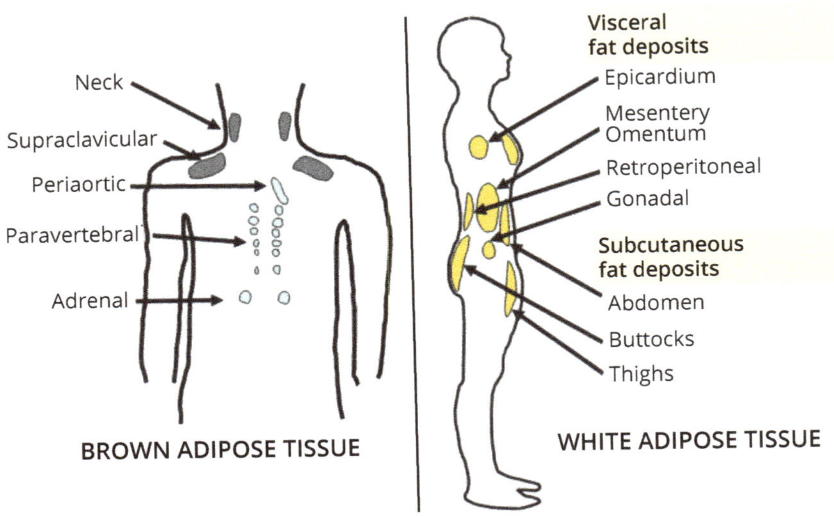

Fig. II-1. Localization of fat in the human body

cells were termed beige adipocytes (Lee Y.H. et al., 2014; Carobbio S. et al., 2019).

This presents another promising avenue for working with adipose tissue: promoting the transformation of white adipocytes into beige ones, which metabolize fat more efficiently. Cryolipolysis — an approach involving localized deep cooling of adipose tissue — may activate this mechanism, encouraging white cells to shift toward a brown-like, heat-generating phenotype (**Fig. II-2**). The transdifferentiation of white adipocytes into beige adipocytes is particularly intriguing for obesity management, making it a focal point for medical research and pharmaceutical development (Moonen M.P.B. et al., 2019).

We highlight this information to underscore that contemporary physiologic approaches targeting subcutaneous fat are well supported by scientific evidence, allowing for effective comparisons and individualized program design. Lafontan emphasizes in his speeches and publications that surgeons performing liposuction and fat transfer with blunt techniques should consider the "fate" of the tissues and cells they manipulate.

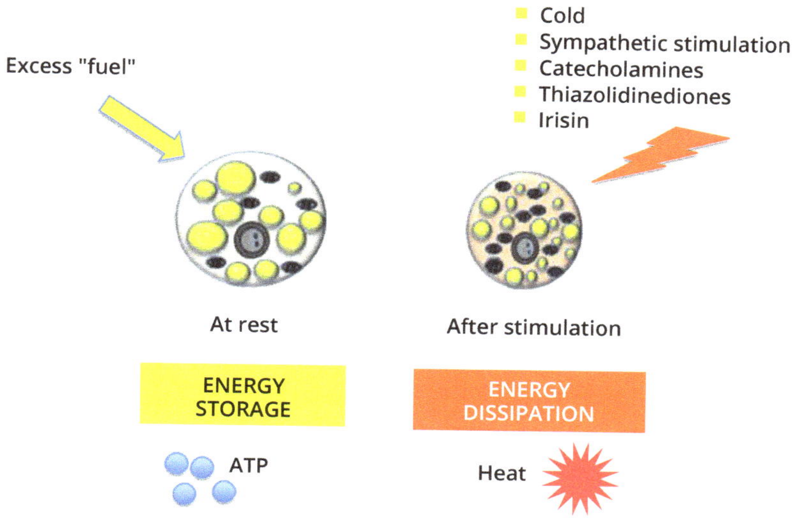

Fig. II-2. Beige adipocytes begin to produce heat after stimulation

1.2. SAT-targeted modalities

Addressing cellulite and localized fat deposits should involve a multifaceted approach, implemented gently yet persistently (Bass L.S., Kaminer M.S., 2020; Khalil S., Galadari H.I., 2024; Menon A. et al., 2024). This can be accomplished through a tailored combination of approaches based on the underlying pathogenesis (**Table II-1**). Key areas for intervention include:

- Normalizing blood circulation and resolving lymphostasis
- Stimulating lipolysis
- Inhibiting lipogenesis
- Restoring fibrous septa in the SAT and dermal layer
- Enhancing muscle function
- Reducing chronic inflammation

Table II-1. Therapeutic objectives and approaches for cellulite and localized fat management

OBJECTIVES	APPROACHES
Stimulating lymphatic and blood circulation Strengthening the vascular wall	• Mesotherapy • Pressotherapy • Mechanovacuum therapy • Massage (manual, device-assisted) • Microcurrent therapy • Carboxytherapy (injectable, topical) • Thalassotherapy
Stimulating lipolysis Suppressing lipogenesis	• Mesotherapy (lipolytics, signal peptides with lipolytic action) • Cryolipolysis • Electrotherapy • Ultrasound therapy • Low-level red/infrared laser (light) therapy (LLLT) • Carboxytherapy • Mechanovacuum therapy • Massage (manual, device-assisted) • Thalassotherapy
Reducing fibrosis	• Ultrasound therapy • RF microneedling • Mesotherapy (defibrotic agents) • Carboxytherapy • Mechanovacuum therapy
Muscle stimulation	• Electromyostimulation • Physical exercise
Improving overall skin condition	• Mesotherapy (eutrophics) • Microcurrent therapy • Carboxytherapy • Thalassotherapy • Mechanovacuum therapy • RF therapy • Massage (manual, device-assisted)
Relieving inflammation	• Microcurrent therapy • LLLT

1.3. Selecting interventions based on the stage of cellulite

At any stage of cellulite and in the presence of localized fat deposits, the most effective approach is a comprehensive correction program that includes the following components:

- A balanced diet
- Targeted physical exercises
- Localized treatment with cosmetic and mesotherapeutic agents
- Manual and device-assisted massage
- Energy-based techniques
- Nutritional supplements

Simply losing weight to eliminate cellulite is ineffective; even with a low-calorie diet, weight loss will occur in all areas except these specific ones. The modern market offers a variety of anti-cellulite products for both internal (tablets, capsules, teas) and external (soaps, gels, creams, scrubs, peels, muds, patches) use. However, these products are effective only when combined with appropriate nutrition and adequate physical activity.

Additionally, mesotherapeutic treatments that enhance microcirculation (blood flow and lymphatic drainage) and stimulate lipolysis, along with various physiotherapeutic approaches targeting the hypodermis and overall skin health, can provide significant benefits.

Stage 1

Gradual changes occur in the affected areas due to stagnation of interstitial fluid, leading to "soft" cellulite. This fluid compresses lymphatic vessels, impairs lymphatic drainage, and causes localized swelling. At this stage, efforts should focus on restoring microcirculation.

Methods:

- Mechanotherapy with a focus on vibration therapy
- Microcurrent therapy
- Carboxytherapy (injectable, topical)
- Mesotherapy to reduce vascular wall permeability
- Cosmetic wraps
- Anti-cellulite cosmetic products

Stage 2

During this stage, fibrous septa of the SAT thicken and become more rigid, resulting in denser SAT that obstructs blood and lymph flow at the capillary level. This leads to more pronounced edema, with the lymphatic system in the affected area functioning at only 30–40% efficiency. The venous system also struggles to drain fluid due to compression of the postcapillary venules, which further increases tissue pressure. Adipocytes undergo hypertrophy due to hypoxia and acidosis, and the skin may leave indentations when pressed, indicating reduced elasticity.

In addition to normalizing microcirculation, priorities include slowing fibrosis and adipocyte hypertrophy and preventing inflammatory progression.

Methods:

- Mechanotherapy (vibration therapy, vacuum therapy)
- Microcurrent therapy
- LLLT
- Carboxytherapy (injectable, topical)
- Mesotherapy (anti-fibrosis support, stimulation of lipolysis, support of the immune status of the skin)
- Cosmetic wraps
- Anti-cellulite cosmetic products

Stage 3

Micronodular stage: liposclerosis develops, leading to the formation of micronodules and the characteristic "orange peel" appearance (often referred to as "hard" cellulite). Symptoms of chronic inflammation are present, resulting in deterioration of dermal structure and skin barrier function. At this stage, destructive approaches that trigger remodeling processes in the SAT and dermis, along with more potent lipolytic agents, can be used.

Methods:

- RF microneedling
- Mesotherapy (stimulation of lipolysis, anti-fibrosis support, normalization of the immune status of the skin)
- Mechanotherapy (vibration therapy, pressotherapy, vacuum therapy)

- Microcurrent therapy
- LLLT
- Carboxytherapy (injectable, topical)
- Cosmetic wraps
- Anti-cellulite cosmetics

Stage 4

Macronodular stage: micronodules increase in number and size, forming macronodules. Surgical intervention may be required.

Methods:

- Liposuction
- Mechanotherapy (vibrotherapy, pressotherapy, vacuum therapy)
- Microcurrent therapy
- LLLT
- Carboxytherapy (injectable, topical)
- Mesotherapy (anti-fibrosis support, stimulation of lipolysis, normalization of the immune status of the skin)
- Cosmetic wraps
- Anti-cellulite cosmetics
- Cosmetic products supporting skin barrier function

Part III

Liposuction

Liposuction (also known as lipoaspiration) is among the most frequently performed procedures in plastic surgery (Shridharani S.M. et al., 2014; Beidas O.E., Gusenoff J.A., 2021). It involves the removal of adipose tissue using a hollow cannula connected to a suction system that creates negative pressure. The cannula is introduced directly into the fat deposit, and the aspirate is removed through the cannula lumen (**Fig. III-1**).

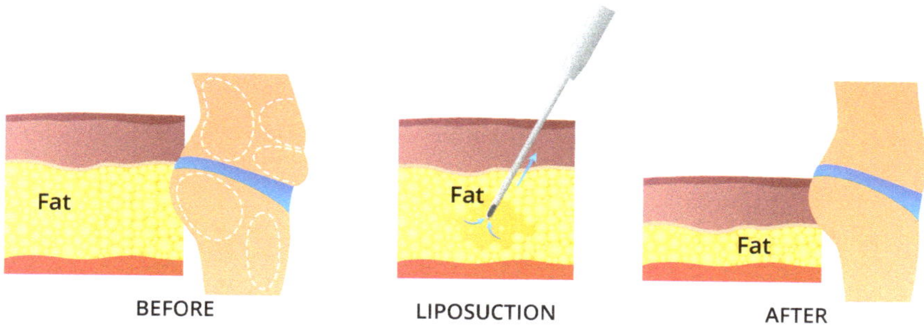

Fig. III-1. Principle of liposuction (Image: Freepik)

Despite its widespread use and significant technical advances, liposuction remains a serious surgical procedure with potential pain, adverse effects, and complications (Wu S. et al., 2020; Pacifico M. et al., 2022).

1.1. Suction-assisted lipectomy (aspiration liposuction)

Traditional suction-assisted liposuction is a relatively traumatic procedure. Mechanical injury to adipose tissue, vessels, nerves, and connective tissue can lead to pain, prolonged bruising, and swelling. The procedure relies on suction-based removal of subcutaneous fat via a cannula, introduced through small incisions.

To reduce trauma and facilitate fat removal, a solution is infiltrated into the treatment area to loosen and separate fat lobules. In the **tumescent technique**, the area is pre-infiltrated with a volume of solution approximately 2-3 times the anticipated lipoaspirate volume.

Today, liposuction approaches that provide controlled exposure to physical modalities are increasingly used. Below, we outline modern liposuction variations and then discuss physical approaches that underpin more conservative body contouring strategies.

1.2. Vibration-assisted liposuction (booster liposuction)

Vibration-assisted liposuction, often described as **booster liposuction**, uses a vibrating cannula to disrupt fat and facilitate aspiration with less manual effort. However, this approach is generally considered more traumatic than traditional suction-assisted lipectomy.

1.3. Radiofrequency-assisted liposuction

One option is **RF-assisted liposuction (RFAL)**, which uses a system with an internal and an external electrode (**Fig. III-2**). An alternating current in the RF range flows between the tip of the hollow, needle-shaped internal electrode — inserted into the fat layer at a defined depth — and the external electrode placed on the skin surface. RF heating promotes softening and liquefaction of subcutaneous fat (Theodorou S.J. et al., 2018). The lipoaspirate is then removed through the internal electrode.

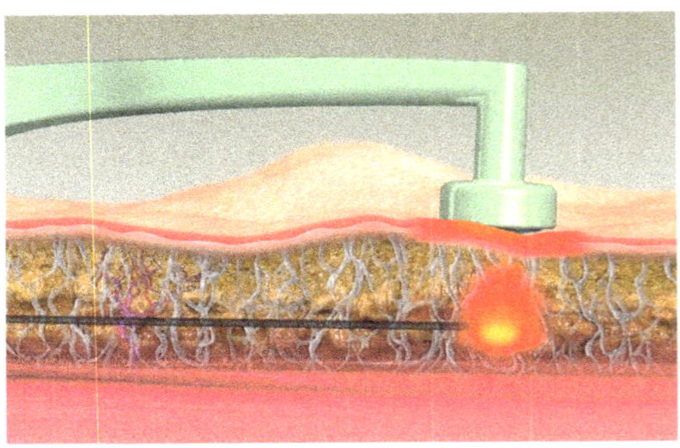

Fig. III-2. RF-assisted liposuction (BodyTite technology; InMode, Israel)

Because heating occurs primarily within the tissue

volume between the two electrodes, lateral spread is limited. This reduces the risk of unintended collateral heating, which can occur with other energy-based approaches — especially those that deliver internal heat (for example, laser-based techniques), where energy can disperse beyond the intended zone.

RF parameters can be calibrated to promote vessel coagulation during adipose-tissue treatment, potentially reducing bleeding and bruising compared with traditional liposuction.

Compared with other liposuction approaches, RFAL offers:

- Minimal invasiveness
- Reduced pain, supporting performance under local anesthesia
- Fewer post-procedural hematomas
- Less swelling
- Shorter recovery time
- Noticeable skin thickening
- Short procedure time

This approach can also be used in facial zones. Because current flows between the internal and external electrodes, primary heating remains relatively confined, reducing thermal exposure to tissue surrounding the internal electrode and helping protect facial nerves in the treatment area.

RFAL is often combined with non-ablative RF therapy, and the sequence matters (Arshakyan V.A., 2020). When RF therapy is performed first, it can soften fibrous septa and promote fat liquefaction, facilitating subsequent aspiration. In this scenario, a substantial portion of the fibrous septa may also be removed during aspiration, thereby reducing postoperative contraction and tissue compaction.

If aspiration is performed first, more septa remain intact. These septa then become targets for subsequent RF exposure, leading to more visible skin contraction. It is also essential to consider that septa may be easier to reduce when the mechanical pressure from fat lobules is lower. After aspiration decreases SAT volume, septa can relax, improving access for RF energy (Han X. et al., 2021).

Electrical approaches in body contouring are discussed in detail in a dedicated chapter (see Part IV, Ch. 2).

1.4. Laser-assisted liposuction

Laser-assisted liposuction involves pretreatment of SAT with laser light followed by tumescent aspiration. Light energy is delivered to the target via an optical fiber, which lowers the risk of superficial burns. Emulsified fat is then removed with suction (laser liposuction) or left to resolve via biologic clearance (**laser lipolysis**).

Beyond treating adipose tissue, laser exposure can also heat the dermis and stimulate fibroblasts to produce extracellular matrix components. This can promote collagen reorganization and dermal thickening. Coagulation of small vessels may reduce blood loss, and the risk of postoperative complications is generally low, supporting a relatively rapid recovery. Procedures typically last no more than an hour.

A limitation is reduced efficiency for large-volume fat removal in a single session. Laser-based approaches are therefore more commonly used in smaller-volume zones, such as the face or submental area.

Light-based approaches for cellulite and localized fat management are discussed in a separate chapter (see Part IV, Ch. 4).

1.5. Ultrasound-assisted liposuction

Ultrasound-assisted liposuction is a gentler option for fat removal. Fat is pre-emulsified primarily via cavitation induced by ultrasound (typically 20-36 kHz) delivered through a probe introduced into the fat layer. Dense surrounding structures — ligaments, fascia, and nerves — are less susceptible to cavitation, helping limit unintended injury. After ultrasound exposure, subcutaneous fat becomes an emulsion that can be aspirated using thin titanium cannulas (2 to 3 mm diameter) with low suction pressure. Lower pressure further reduces the risk of skin trauma and injury to nearby vessels and nerves.

Advantages include:

- Minimal blood loss
- Ability to remove substantial fat volume in a single procedure
- More even fat removal, reducing contour irregularities
- Faster and easier recovery

Ultrasound-assisted liposuction does not coagulate vessels, so skin tightening is typically limited (Atieh B. et al., 2025). Sound-based approaches for cellulite and localized fat management are discussed in a separate chapter (see Part IV, Ch. 3).

1.6. Treatment of post-liposuction skin irregularities

Liposuction can occasionally lead to visible contour irregularities due to uneven fat removal, negatively affecting outcomes and patient satisfaction. This has increased interest in effective and safe corrective options.

Recently, injectable formulations that stimulate collagen production have attracted attention. One example is calcium hydroxyapatite (CaHA), which is widely used in aesthetic medicine, including wrinkle correction and overall skin quality improvement.

Available data suggest CaHA may help address post-liposuction irregularities. In particular, diluted (1:1) or hyperdiluted (1:2) CaHA injections have been associated with a statistically significant reduction in the number and depth of depressions, along with a trend toward improved skin elasticity (Guida S. et al., 2025). Proposed mechanisms include fibroblast stimulation, leading to increased collagen production and reinforcement of the skin structure (Nowag B. et al., 2023).

Evidence remains early, and larger studies with longer follow-up are needed to confirm durability and refine protocols. Still, current findings suggest that biostimulatory fillers such as CaHA may offer an effective and safe option for post-liposuction surface irregularities.

Key considerations include:

- **CaHA concentration selection** based on depression depth and severity, with higher concentrations for deeper defects and lower concentrations for superficial irregularities (Guida S. et al., 2025)
- **Injection technique selection**, with the "crosswise" technique described as helpful for even product distribution (Guida S. et al., 2025)
- **Combination strategies** to enhance outcomes, including pairing CaHA with RF microneedling or HIFU-assisted SMAS lifting and tightening (Casabona G., Pereira G., 2017)

While this option shows promise, additional research is required to validate long-term outcomes and define optimal protocols (Guida S. et al., 2025).

Despite advances in surgical liposuction, procedural risk remains meaningful. In obesity — a complex condition often accompanied by severe systemic disease — surgery may be necessary. However, when the concern is localized fat deposits or cellulite, which are typically considered aesthetic issues, a longer but substantially lower-risk approach is generally preferable (Kennedy J. et al., 2015; Alizadeh Z. et al., 2016).

A trend toward minimally invasive and conservative body contouring continues to grow. Notably, significant progress has been made in non-surgical device-based approaches. These strategies can stimulate lipolysis and support dermal and hypodermal remodeling, helping with tissue tightening after volume reduction. Combining device-assisted massage, injectables, cosmetics, and supportive garments within an anti-cellulite program can meaningfully increase the likelihood of achieving the desired outcome.

Part IV

Body-contouring devices and procedures

A central component of an anti-cellulite aesthetic program is the use of devices that deliver physical energy to deeper skin layers. While many options exist, they share a common capability: activating physiologic processes that reduce SAT volume. At the same time, superficial skin layers are either unaffected or only minimally disrupted, thereby substantially lowering the risk. Unlike injectable procedures, these approaches can treat larger areas without allergic reactions or other adverse effects associated with injected substances. And unlike cosmetic products that mainly act on the surface, physical energy can reach deeper tissues.

Depending on the primary mechanism, these approaches can be grouped into five categories:

1. Mechanical
2. Electrical
3. Light
4. Sound
5. Temperature

Combined technologies also exist and incorporate more than one mechanism. For example, RF microneedling creates multiple skin punctures with needle electrodes while delivering alternating RF current. Other combinations are also used and are discussed in the relevant sections.

Chapter 1
Mechanical technologies

One of the oldest and most accessible ways to influence the body is massage. In general, massage involves mechanical action on the skin using hands or dedicated tools. Techniques vary and may include:

- Pressure (static at a point or dynamic across multiple areas)
- Tapping
- Vibration
- Compression and decompression
- Stretching
- Kneading
- Stroking

Massage techniques have evolved over centuries, based on observations and practical experience passed down through generations. It was not until the 20th century, with advances in medical engineering, that massage progressed substantially. New devices improved control over applied force and exposure time and enabled the combination of mechanical action with other inputs, such as light and temperature.

A dedicated field, **skin mechanobiology**, has since emerged. It focuses on the biomechanical properties of dermal tissues and how cells respond to external mechanical forces. This research has reshaped how we think about the skin's role in massage: the skin is not merely a passive conduit relaying signals to deeper, damaged tissues. It actively participates and can undergo structural change. This opens additional opportunities to use massage for skin rejuvenation and to address a range of aesthetic concerns, including body contouring.

Today, massage techniques are an essential component of aesthetic care aimed at improving skin structure and function. However, to achieve durable, clinically meaningful results, dedicated tools are often needed to reliably reach different depths and address multiple targets simultaneously. To emphasize these clinical capabilities, massage performed with devices is increasingly referred to as **mechanotherapy**.

1.1. Mechanotherapy: molecular and cellular mechanisms

External mechanical forces can deform the skin, altering its three-dimensional structure (**Fig. IV-1-1**). Both the extracellular matrix and the cells themselves undergo deformation. This triggers cellular processes that affect function and lead to tissue-level structural remodeling.

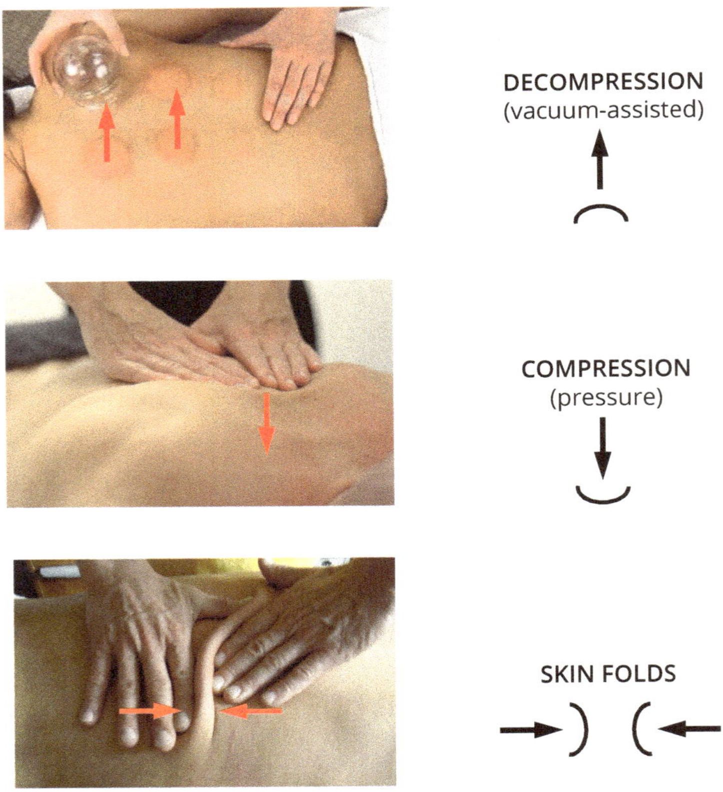

Fig. IV-1-1. Skin deformation during massage

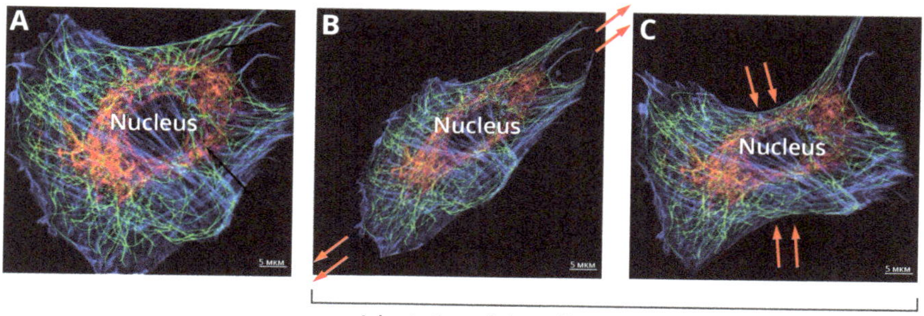

Fig. IV-1-2. Fibroblast cytoskeleton (fluorescence micrograph): microtubules (green), intermediate filaments (red).
A — fibroblast at rest; B, C — cytoskeletal and shape changes in the fibroblast under external deforming forces (adapted from Pollard T.D., Goldman R.D., 2018; CC BY)

1.1.1. Cell cytoskeleton and extracellular matrix

Every living cell contains a protein framework known as the cytoskeleton (**Fig. IV-1-2**) (Pollard T.D., Goldman R.D., 2018). The cytoskeleton maintains cell shape at rest and is essential for movement, whether the entire cell migrates or parts of the cell capture and release substances from the surrounding environment (Pollard T.D., 2016). When the external environment changes mechanically, the cytoskeleton deforms: the cell may stretch globally, or specific regions may distort.

Cytoskeletal changes activate biochemical pathways that help the cell adapt to its environment. When fibroblasts undergo prolonged stretching, they increase fibrillar protein synthesis, forming a three-dimensional network. The fibroblast attaches to this fiber network and senses changes in tension because its internal cytoskeleton also shifts configuration (**Fig. IV-1-3**). To improve the skin's resistance to stretch, fibroblasts reinforce the tissue by producing new structural proteins, including collagen. This is one way skin adapts to increased mechanical load (Humphrey J.D. et al., 2014).

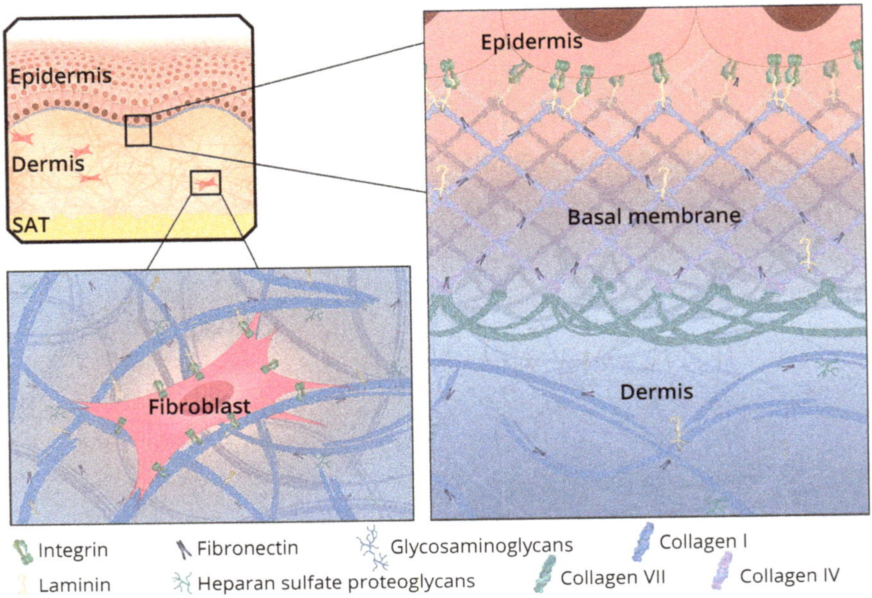

Fig. IV-1-3. Major structural molecules of the skin extracellular matrix (adapted from Pfisterer K. et al., 2021; CC BY)

1.1.2. PIEZO channels: cellular mechanoreceptors

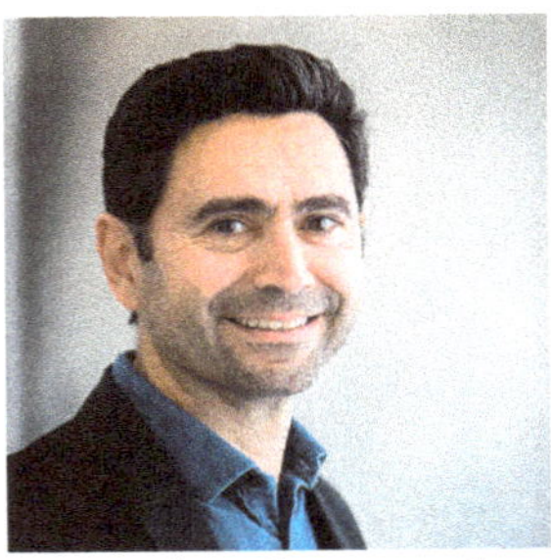

Dr. Ardem Patapoutian

Beyond the cytoskeleton, the cell's outer layer — the cell membrane — can also participate in mechanosensing. The membrane is a lipid bilayer, a thin, flexible film. Under mechanical load, it bends, and its lateral tension changes. Even small changes can be enough to alter the conformation of proteins embedded in the membrane. For many proteins, this has no functional impact. However, some cells contain specialized proteins that are highly sensitive to membrane deformation.

These proteins form ion channels. They were described in 2010 by American molecular biologist and neuroscientist Ardem Patapoutian, who named them PIEZO, from the Greek word πιέζω (piezo), meaning "press" or "compression." For this discovery, Dr. Patapoutian received

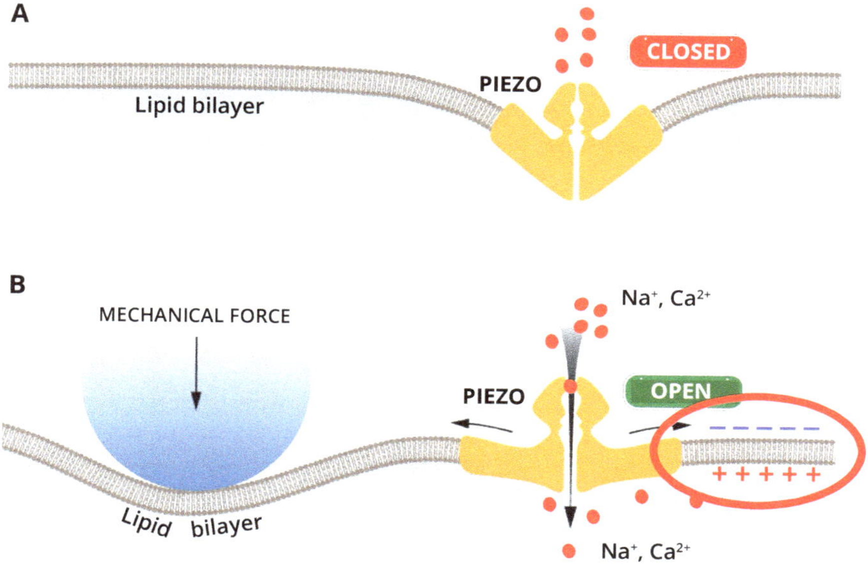

Fig. IV-1-4. PIEZO channels: mechanically gated ion channels

the 2021 Nobel Prize in Physiology or Medicine (Kefauver J.M. et al., 2020).

Typically, PIEZO channels are closed; hence, they are also called mechanically gated or stretch-activated channels (**Fig. IV-1-4**). When the membrane near one of these proteins is stretched by external force, the protein deforms, and the channel opens (Parpaite T., Coste B., 2017).

1.1.3. Tactile receptors: mechanoreceptors of the skin

PIEZO channels are present in endings of sensory (afferent) nerve fibers that respond to mechanical stimuli such as touch, pressure, and stretch. These specialized sensors are collectively called mechanoreceptors.

Mechanoreceptors in different organs are typically named for their function. Baroreceptors in vessel walls, the heart, and the bladder detect fluid pressure. Proprioceptors in muscles and joints respond to stretch and help coordinate movement. Vestibular receptors detect head motion and are critical for spatial orientation. Tactile receptors mediate skin sensitivity (Abraira V.E., Ginty D.D., 2013).

Although mechanoreceptors differ in structure across tissues, the core principles of detection and signal transmission are similar. The sequence can be represented as follows:

1. When the membrane is mechanically deformed, a PIEZO channel opens, allowing positively charged ions (such as Ca^{2+} and Na^{+}) to enter the cell (**Fig. IV-1-4B**).
2. On the inner side of the membrane, where negative ions predominate at rest, incoming positive ions reverse the local charge from "–" to "+". At rest, the membrane is negative inside and positive outside. When channels open and positive ions flow inward, polarity briefly shifts — this phenomenon called membrane depolarization (Ridone P. et al., 2019).
3. The depolarized region becomes the origin of a depolarization wave — a nerve impulse — that propagates. In a sensory neuron, the impulse travels from the mechanoreceptor along the axon. Eventually, excitation reaches the next neuron and the signal is relayed onward (**Fig. IV-1-5**).
4. The impulse ultimately reaches the brain (**Fig. IV-1-6**), where information is processed, and an appropriate response is selected. Commands then travel down motor neurons to their terminals. This triggers the release of signaling molecules that affect other skin cells, including immunocytes, endotheliocytes, keratinocytes, fibroblasts, and adipocytes. Each cell type responds to specific signals in a cell-specific way.

This is a broad, simplified outline of how external mechanical forces can influence skin structure, where **"deformation" is the key concept**.

- **Deformation of the extracellular matrix** affects the cytoskeleton and initiates biochemical processes within the cell; fibroblasts provide a clear example of direct detection.
- **Deformation of the cell membrane** can open PIEZO channels in tactile receptors, activating them and sending signals to

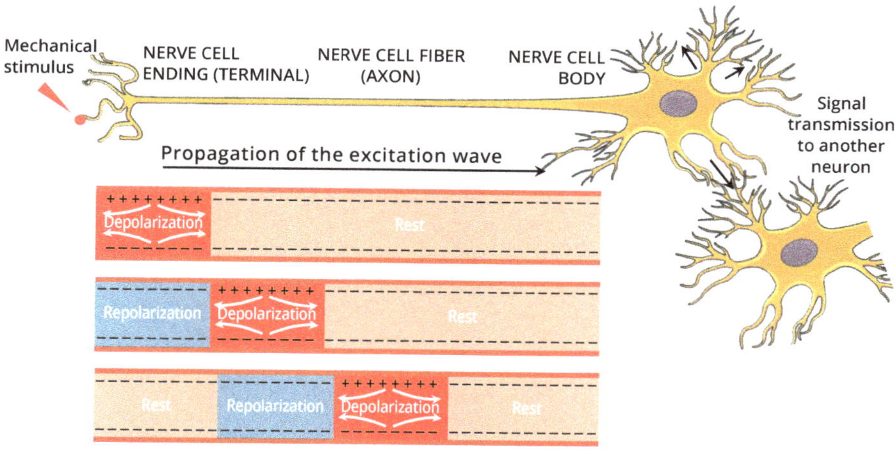

Fig. IV-1-5. Propagation of an excitation wave (impulse) along a nerve fiber

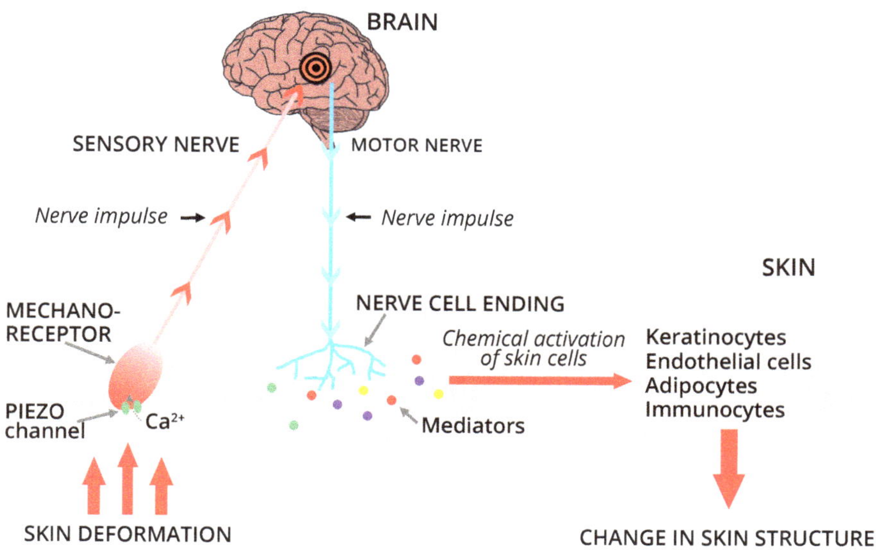

Fig. IV-1-6. Principles of skin mechanosensitivity

the CNS via sensory nerve fibers. Commands are then returned to skin cells via chemical mediators released at motor nerve terminals. This pathway is referred to as indirect sensitivity.

Ultimately, all skin cells participate — directly or indirectly — in the response to mechanical forces and contribute to structural reorganization. The specific nature of the reaction depends on mechanical parameters such as force, duration, and direction (perpendicular to the skin vs. parallel to the surface).

1.2. Mechanotherapy technologies: variants and effects

Mechanical effects on the skin can be **constant** (often referred to as mechanical stress) or **variable**, such as those produced by mechanical vibrations (vibration therapy).

Mechanical stresses can also be classified by whether pressure is applied **above atmospheric pressure** (pressotherapy) or **below** it (vacuum therapy).

1.2.1. Manual massage

Manual massage is the simplest and most widely used form of mechanotherapy. Its effectiveness largely depends on the practitioner's skill and the techniques applied.

The clinical benefits of manual massage are commonly attributed to several mechanisms:

- Release of physiologically active, histamine-like substances with vasodilatory effects. Their action is relatively prolonged and can extend into deeper layers, influencing muscle tissue and improving soft-tissue nutrition.
- Improved lymphatic flow, supporting restoration of cutaneous homeostasis.
- Increased muscle tone contributes to smoother, firmer-looking skin.

1.2.2. Compression therapy

Compression therapy refers to techniques that apply pressure to the skin. In skincare and aesthetic medicine, pressotherapy and Shiatsu are among the most widely used approaches.

Pressotherapy

Pressotherapy, also known as pneumatic massage or air-compression therapy, uses inflatable cuffs (leg or arm sleeves) that fill with air and rhythmically compress and release, simulating elements of manual massage. This approach improves circulation, supports lymphatic drainage, reduces swelling and soreness, and can speed muscle recovery by promoting fluid shift and the clearance of metabolic byproducts.

A compression-decompression cycle during a session typically lasts 30 s to 2 min. When cuff pressure is released, vasodilation occurs, increasing blood flow to the skin, subcutaneous tissue, and muscles.

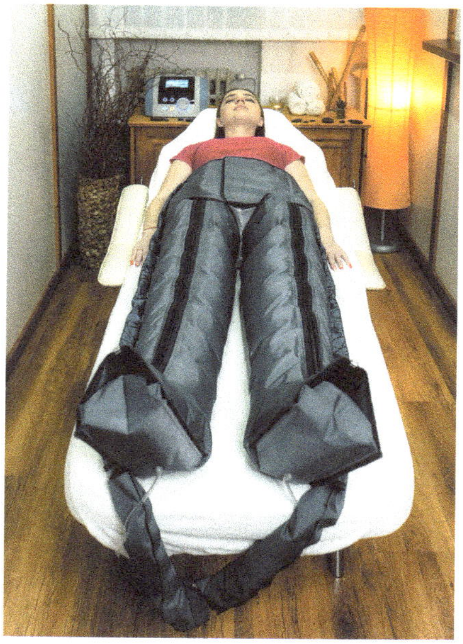

Fig. IV-1-7. Pressotherapy session (Photo: Freepik)

In aesthetics, pressotherapy is primarily used for its effects on circulation and lymphatic flow (**Fig. IV-1-7**). The goal is to support blood and lymphatic circulation, which is critical for cellulite management. Pneumatic compression systems that add heat are available and used to accelerate metabolic processes. In addition, during pneumatic massage, topical preparations with lipolytic ingredients may be applied (Ptaszek B. et al., 2024).

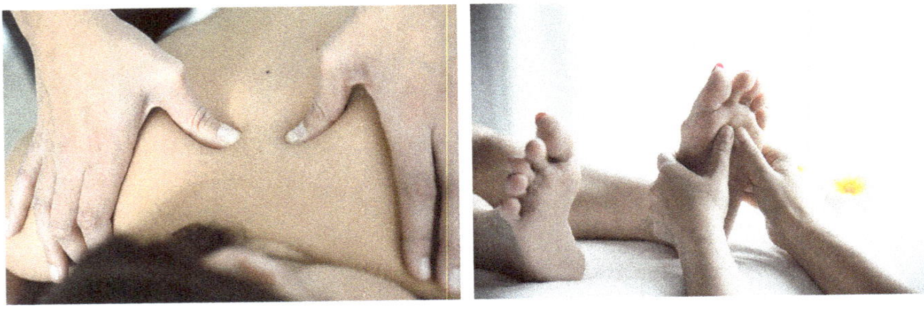

Fig. IV-1-8. Shiatsu massage (Photo: Freepik)

Shiatsu massage

Shiatsu is a Japanese therapeutic technique based on principles of traditional Chinese medicine. It involves applying pressure to specific points on the body to reduce pain, refresh the skin, relieve stress, and address or help prevent a range of complaints (**Fig. IV-1-8**). During Shiatsu, pressure is applied with the thumb perpendicular to the body, without sliding, until tissues in the treated area soften. The approach resembles reflexology, which focuses on biologically active points with a high density of nerve endings.

Although Shiatsu devices are available, many people feel that mechanical massagers do not match the effect of skilled hands. Early on, these devices may feel noticeably pleasant; however, after a couple of weeks, receptors can adapt to repetitive motion, reducing perceived benefit. To reduce habituation, modern massage devices often offer multiple operating modes, although this does not fully solve the issue.

A well-known Shiatsu-style foot massage system is produced by Marutaka (Japan). It uses three rollers operating in four mixed directions, creating a sensation similar to massage by two strong hands. With three modes (relaxing, intensive, and speed), rollers rotate at 30–48 revolutions per minute. Adjusting modes and settings can help reduce habituation.

While mechanical massage can feel intense, manual Shiatsu can be uncomfortable as well. If you are fatigued, Shiatsu may leave you feeling refreshed and energized. Conversely, if you think about being over-stimulated, it may help you relax or even fall asleep. This effect is associated with increased circulation and stimulation of multiple nerve endings in the feet, supporting restoration of physiologic balance.

In addition to an acupuncture-style foot massage, the system may include ankle massage and elevation features, as well as an inflatable cushion that adapts the massage surface to different foot heights.

1.2.3. Vibration therapy

Vibromassage involves low-frequency (20–200 Hz) mechanical vibrations with varying amplitudes and directions. Because it is difficult to manually maintain a stable vibration pattern for extended periods, devices are used to do so.

Consider what happens to the skin during vibrotherapy. Strong vibrations create extracellular fluid movement. On the one hand, this can enhance nutrient delivery to cells; on the other, it can support the removal of metabolic byproducts. This is particularly relevant when microcirculation is impaired, and tissue congestion is present, as in cellulite, where enlarged fat lobules compress vessels and lymphatic ducts.

Vibration therapy acts not only by moving extracellular fluid but also by influencing living skin cells through tissue deformation (Kim D., Kwon S., 2020). In the treated area, vessels and capillaries dilate, improving blood flow and enhancing the delivery of oxygen and nutrients. Lymphatic ducts also dilate, supporting clearance of metabolic byproducts.

Vibrotherapy can be especially helpful for cellulite because it reduces congestion and swelling that develop when enlarged fat lobules compress capillaries and lymphatic ducts. Thermographic data also suggest that both single and repeated vibrotherapy sessions can increase skin temperature in cellulite-prone zones (**Fig. IV-1-9**), consistent with improved cutaneous blood flow and, potentially, better nutrient delivery to the treated area. Notably, longer-term effects observed after a course of treatments may be particularly relevant for cellulite management, although further research is needed to clarify the relationships among vibrotherapy, gynoid lipodystrophy, and skin temperature (Pilch W. et al., 2019). While other skin layers can benefit as well, the most pronounced changes typically occur in the SAT, where fat lobules are located.

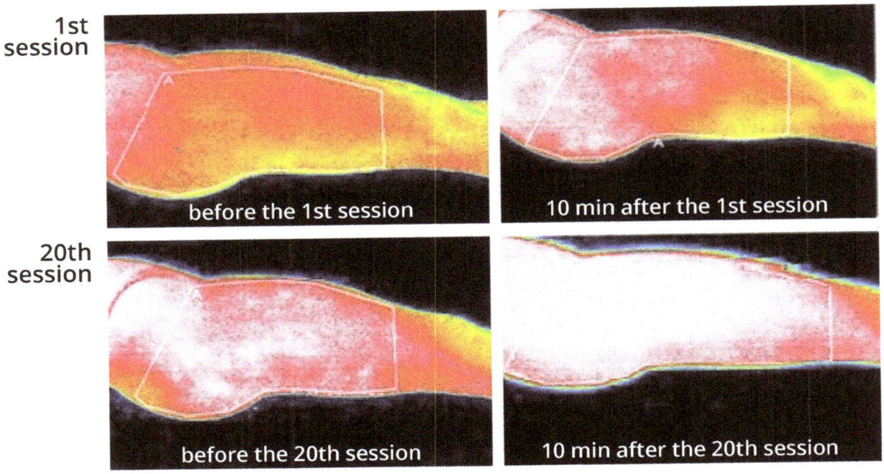

Fig. IV-1-9. Thermograms of a patient's lateral thigh with cellulite: before and after vibration treatment (adapted from Pilch W. et al., 2019; CC BY)

1.2.4. Vacuum therapy (decompression)

Traditional vacuum therapy is rarely used as a standalone approach. More often, it is combined with other modalities such as vibration or pressure (see Part IV, section 1.3). Still, several aesthetic approaches rely on negative pressure applied to the skin.

For example, vacuum massage is sometimes used to improve breast shape. The procedure uses a system with a pump and cup-shaped pads. The massage increases blood circulation in breast tissue, and nipple stimulation is proposed to support estrogen production, a hormone that influences breast development. In addition, the approach may tone muscles overlying the breast, producing a mild lifting effect.

One perceived advantage is rapid visible change: after a single session, breast size may increase by 1–2 cup sizes due to improved blood flow. However, maintaining this effect typically requires daily sessions. Rapid enlargement can also stretch the skin, potentially contributing to the development of stretch marks.

1.3. Combined mechanotherapy

Modern body-contouring approaches may combine multiple mechanical modalities to reduce fat volume and tighten the skin. Below are examples.

1.3.1. Vibrovacuum therapy: decompression + vibration

Vibrovacuum therapy combines localized vacuum decompression (up to 50 kPa) with vibration (10–70 Hz). The handpiece creates negative pressure beneath a dome while simultaneously generating vibration and transmitting it into tissue (**Fig. IV-1-10**).

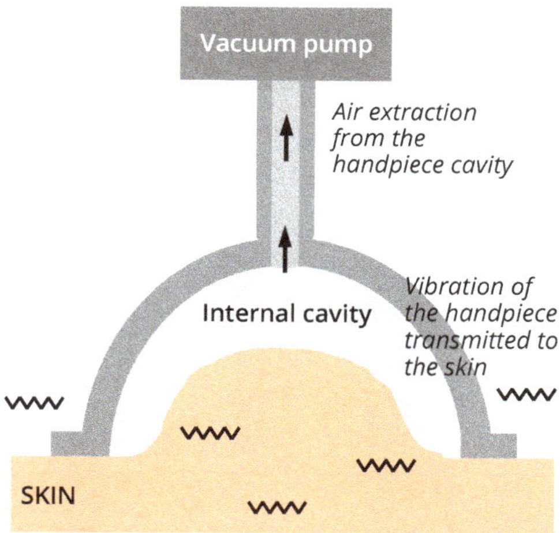

Fig. IV-1-10. Vibrovacuum therapy: decompression + vibration

This approach dilates skin vessels, improving microcirculation and lymph flow across larger areas. As a result, swelling decreases and excess fluid, along with metabolic byproducts, is cleared. Skin quality may improve, with tissue appearing firmer and more elastic — an essential effect in laxity after weight loss or childbirth.

In addition, vibrovacuum massage increases circulation to muscles and ligaments, supporting metabolism and nutrient delivery. This can strengthen muscles and improve tolerance to physical load. In overworked muscles, tone elevation and soreness may gradually decrease, supporting faster recovery.

1.3.2. Vacuum-roller massage: decompression + kneading

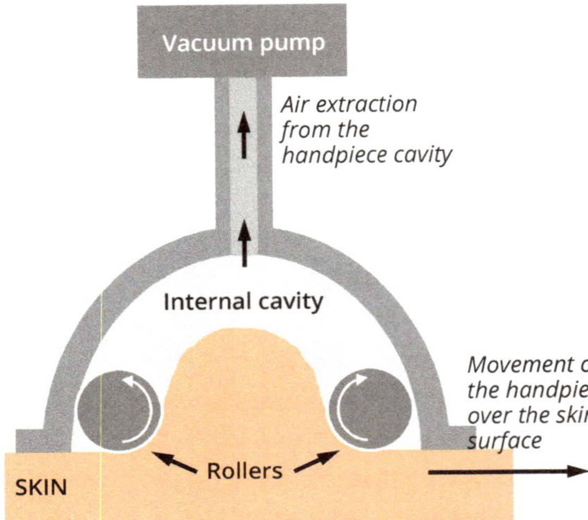

Fig. IV-1-11. Vacuum–roller massage: decompression + stretching

This approach uses a dome-shaped handpiece connected to a vacuum pump and equipped with rollers (**Fig. IV-1-11**). The pump removes air, creating mild negative pressure beneath the handpiece (decompression). The skin is gently lifted as rollers rotate, compressing its edges. The handpiece moves across the surface, systematically treating adjacent zones. After a course of sessions, increases in skin thickness and smoother contours may be observed.

Vacuum-roller massage, widely known as Endermologie®, was introduced in the early 1990s by Louis-Paul Gauthier. The concept emerged after he suffered a serious accident and required extensive massage. He developed and patented a device for rehabilitation massage and, during trials, observed that it could reduce swelling and improve skin texture by tightening, firming, and smoothing the skin while decreasing fat deposits. The technology became widely known as LPG, an abbreviation derived from his name. The first LPG systems appeared in 1994. In 2013, the Ergolift handpiece was introduced, incorporating a micromotor that enables treatment in two dimensions: vertical (perpendicular to the skin surface) and horizontal (parallel to the surface). This supports three-dimensional mechanostimulation of the skin, both at the surface and below it.

Vacuum-roller massage may be used for alimentary-constitutional obesity, cellulite, uneven skin texture (including wrinkles, laxity, folds, and scars), and minor muscle and tendon injuries, supporting restoration of muscle tone and skin turgor.

The combined approaches described above also have meaningful limitations related to vacuum exposure. Contraindications for vacuum massage include:

- Vascular fragility
- Varicosity and impaired circulation
- Tendency to hematoma formation
- Increased pain sensitivity

1.3.3. Vibrocompression therapy

Vibrocompression therapy combines vibration with compression and can address some limitations of other approaches. In aesthetic medicine, this technology is known as Compressive Microvibration®, delivered using the Endospheres Therapy® system (Phenix Group, Italy), which helped establish a new trend in massage-based care.

The vibrocompression handpiece is cylindrical and covered with multiple silicone spheres (**Fig. IV-1-12**). The spheres are mounted on longitudinal axes and rotate freely on contact, allowing smooth gliding over the treatment area. The cylinder itself rotates around its central axis.

During a session, the practitioner applies pressure as they move the vibrating cylinder. Compression and vibration are transmitted

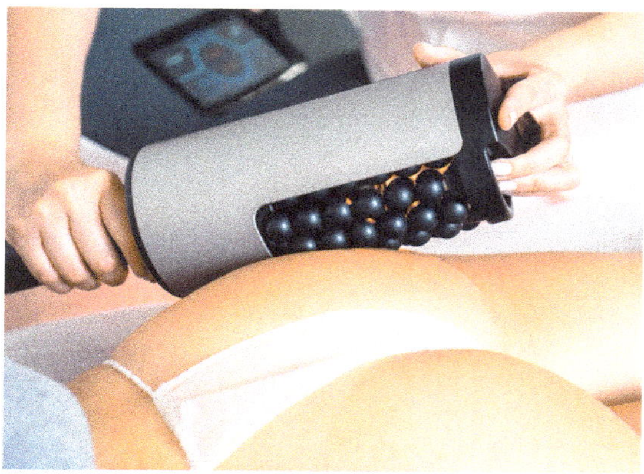

Fig. IV-1-12. Vibrocompression massage handpiece (Photo: Vladimka production/ Shutterstock)

through the spheres, which contact the skin sequentially as the cylinder rolls. Because the force from each sphere is small, compression and microvibration at each contact point are gentle and typically comfortable, without pain. The approach does not injure the skin and does not usually cause bruising.

Multiple contact points also create a pronounced cumulative effect within the treatment zone:

- Rhythmic compression combined with multiple microvibration points supports circulation and improves lymph flow.
- Microvibration may help "soften" fat deposits and support lipolysis.
- Soothing effects may occur.
- Muscle spasm and tension may decrease.
- After a course of therapy (6–12 sessions, 2–3 per week), skin quality may improve, with tighter and smoother skin as connective tissue remodels.

Some contemporary systems also include embedded LEDs that emit red light at 650–660 nm. This low-intensity red light is proposed to help normalize immune cell function and may be helpful for reactive, hypersensitive skin.

Vibrocompression therapy has been used **in several areas**:

1. **Skincare and aesthetic medicine** (**Fig. IV-1-13**):
   - Excess fat deposits in stages 1–2
   - Gynoid lipodystrophy (cellulite at any stage)
   - Skin laxity and low turgor
   - Swelling and congestion
   - Preparation for cosmetic surgery and subsequent rehabilitation
2. **Sports medicine:**
   - Lactic acid buildup in muscles ("clogged" muscles)
   - Muscle spasm
   - Improving muscle microcirculation before competition
3. **Wellness medicine:**
   - General strengthening massage
   - Symptoms of heavy and fatigued legs

CHANGES IN THE DERMAL MATRIX — CHANGES IN THE SAT

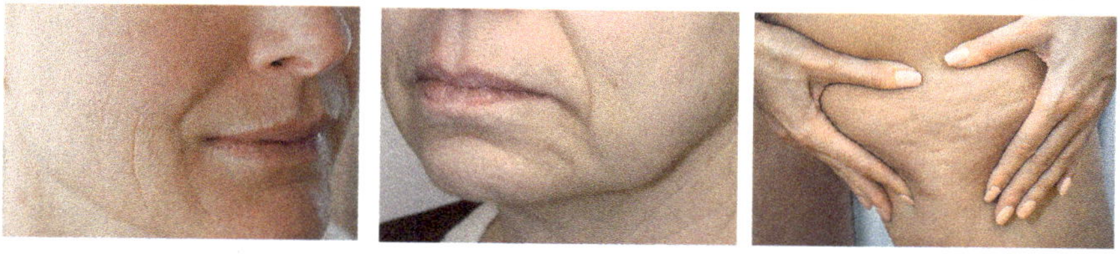

Changes in the dermal matrix

- Low skin turgor
- Superficial and mid-deep wrinkles

- Sagging
- Ptosis
- Deep wrinkles and grooves

Changes in the SAT

- Increased volume in areas of localized fat
- Bumpy texture
- Swelling
- Occasional cyanosis

Fig. IV-1-13. Aesthetic concerns addressed by massage therapy

Like any therapeutic intervention, vibrocompression therapy has **contraindications**, including:

- Cancer in remission for up to 5 years
- Pregnancy
- Acute infectious diseases
- Exacerbation of chronic conditions
- Hyperthermia (elevated body temperature)
- Hemophilia
- Epilepsy
- Hepatic, renal, cardiac, or respiratory insufficiency in the decompensation stage
- Extensive skin disorders

1.4. Future of mechanotherapy

Mechanotherapy is a specialized area within cosmetic dermatology and aesthetic medicine with considerable promise. Advances in computer science, engineering, and biomedical research have driven its growth.

A key breakthrough was the discovery of PIEZO channels in mechanoreceptors, which improved our understanding of how skin detects mechanical forces and communicates those signals to the CNS. It was later shown that PIEZO channels are present in non-excitable cells as well, where calcium influx can trigger a distinct range of Ca^{2+}-dependent biochemical pathways, including genome-related signaling, with cell-type-specific effects.

For example, PIEZO channels are thought to regulate epithelial cell density on the basal membrane. When cells become crowded, membrane deformation can open PIEZO channels, and ion influx may trigger cell death or detachment from the basal membrane (Gudipaty S.A. et al., 2017; Piddini E., 2017).

PIEZO-like channels have also been identified in mesenchymal stem cells and may influence fate decisions and differentiation pathways (He L. et al., 2018; Huang Z. et al., 2023). They are also present in adipocytes, where they may respond to changes in membrane tension associated with fat gain or loss, contributing to adipose tissue remodeling (Miron T.R. et al., 2022; Catalán V. et al., 2024).

Overall, the discovery of PIEZO channels has opened a broad area of research that remains largely unexplored. One point is clear: mechanical action on skin can produce meaningful biologic effects. To ensure these effects are beneficial, it is essential to understand what is being done and why.

For this reason, mechanotherapy should be approached thoughtfully — not merely as an anti-cellulite or remodeling massage, but as a substantial intervention for both skin and the body as a whole. To avoid adverse outcomes and achieve desired results, it is critical to control exposure parameters and technique. The idea that "stronger, longer, and more frequent" always means "better" is a misconception. Following established protocols and manufacturer guidelines is essential, as reputable manufacturers base their recommendations on research findings.

Chapter 2
Electrical technologies

Methods of electrotherapy that use electric current as the main therapeutic factor have been part of body contouring protocols for many years. They differ in how the current is delivered into the tissues and in their parameter settings, with each technique targeting specific problems associated with cellulite and localized fat deposits.

- **High-energy techniques** based on radiofrequency currents (**RF therapy**) are applied to decrease SAT volume, improve skin firmness, and increase tissue thickness.
- **Low-intensity techniques** aim to enhance blood flow and lymphatic drainage (**microcurrent therapy**), activate lipolysis (**electrolipolysis**), and provoke muscle contractions (**electro-myostimulation** and **magnetic myostimulation**).

2.1. Basic characteristics of electric current

Electric current is the orderly, directional movement of charged particles such as electrons and ions. **Current strength (current)** describes how much electric charge passes through a conductor's cross-section each second. It is measured in amperes (A).

For charged particles to start moving, a driving force is needed. This force is created by an **electric field**, in which charges drift in opposite directions: positively charged particles move toward the negative pole. In contrast, negatively charged particles move toward the positive pole.

Voltage (potential difference) is a scalar quantity that reflects the work the field performs when a unit positive charge is moved from one point to another. Voltage is measured in volts (V).

In electrotherapy, an electric field is created in the selected area of the body, causing charges in the local soft tissues to move in an organized way — i.e., producing an electric current. The magnitude and direction of that current are determined by how the voltage is delivered.

- If the field's polarity stays the same (constant voltage), the current flows in a single direction. This is **direct (galvanic) current (DC)**.
- If the polarity switches back and forth at a set rate (alternating voltage), the current reverses direction at the same rate. This is **alternating current (AC)**. The **AC frequency** is the number of direction changes per second and is measured in hertz (Hz).

Current persists only while the driving voltage is present. If the driving force is applied without interruption, the current is **continuous**. If it switches on and off, the current is discontinuous (pulsed). Pulses may have different waveforms — rectangular, triangular, exponential, or half-sine (**Fig. IV-2-1**). Pulsed operation also has a **pulse frequency** (the number of pulses per second), which should not be confused with AC frequency.

When the driving force remains present, but its parameters vary — such as amplitude or frequency — the current is described as modulated. With amplitude modulation, the current's strength changes over time; with frequency modulation, the frequency varies (**Fig. IV-2-2**).

Electric current can be alternating, pulsed, and modulated at the same time. In these situations, it is described using both the alternating-current frequency and the pulse repetition rate, along with

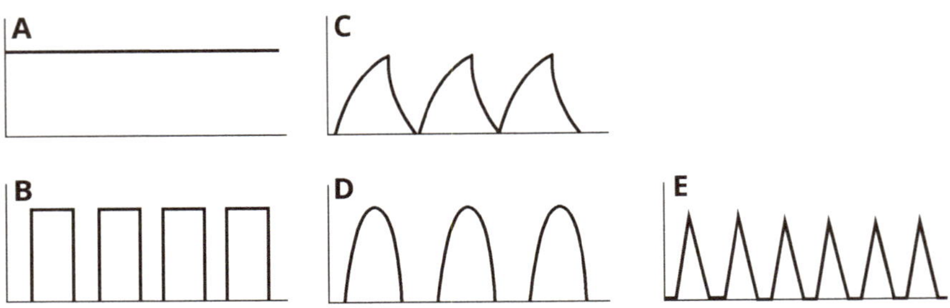

Fig. IV-2-1. Current modes: A — continuous current; B — rectangular pulses; C — exponential pulses; D — half-sinusoidal pulses; E — triangular pulses

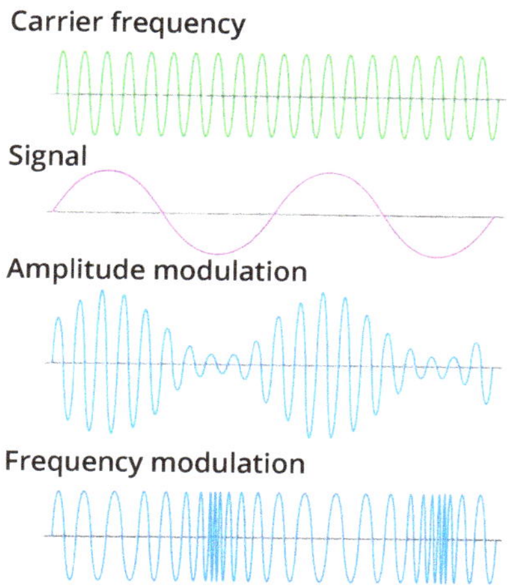

Fig. IV-2-2. Types of modulations

the modulation type. **Fig. IV-2-3** illustrates a modulated current pattern used in diadynamic therapy*.

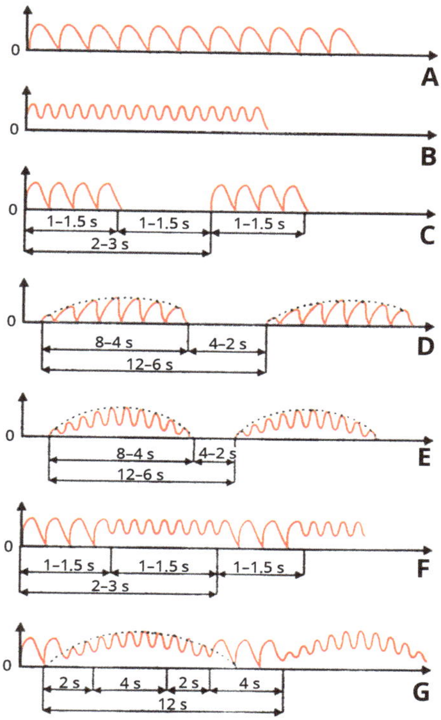

Fig. IV-2-3. Examples of modulated diadynamic currents: A — one-half-period continuous; B — two-half-period; C — one-half-period rhythmic; D — one-half-period; E two-half-period; F — modulated by short periods; G —modulated by long periods

* Diadynamic therapy is an electrotherapy method based on pulses of direct current delivered at 50–100 Hz. The technique was introduced in 1946 by the French dentist P. Bernard, who called these waveforms "diadynamic" currents (also known as Bernard currents). It was originally applied for anesthesia, but later work showed that diadynamic currents also affect tissue perfusion. With transverse electrode placement, capillary blood flow improves and the tone of spasmodic vessels decreases; with longitudinal placement, blood flow may increase two- to threefold. The beneficial effects of this therapy on wound healing, tissue regeneration, and inflammatory processes are well documented.

2.2. Interaction of electric current and biological tissue

In the human body, most charge carriers are found in water-based environments such as blood and extracellular fluid. When an electric field is applied, these particles begin to drift, creating an electric current within the tissues. The effects depend on two main factors: how readily the tissue conducts electricity (its electrical conductivity) and the characteristics of the applied current.

2.2.1. Tissue conductivity

Several terms are commonly used to describe how tissues respond to electric current and to explain clinical effects:

- **Dielectric properties** describe a material's ability to store and hold electric charge when exposed to an alternating electric field.
- **Electrical resistance** reflects how strongly a tissue opposes current flow; it is measured in ohms (Ω).
- **Electrical conductivity** is the inverse of resistance: the higher the conductivity, the more easily current passes through the material.

Multiple factors influence electrical conductivity in tissues:

- **Water content (hydration):** better-hydrated tissues conduct more effectively.
- **Availability of free charge carriers**: in living tissues, these are mainly ions.
- **Tissue structure**: conductivity is shaped by features such as tissue density, the amount of extracellular fluid, the proportion of poorly soluble components (e.g., fat and keratin), and the presence of structural elements (including connective-tissue and nerve fibers).
- **Temperature**: conductivity generally increases with temperature because ions move more easily.

- **Current parameters**: resistance to direct or low-frequency current is mainly determined by the tissue's physical and chemical composition; prolonged exposure to high-intensity currents can lead to heating and burns. With high-frequency currents, apparent resistance usually falls due to dielectric behavior (notably capacitive effects) and the skin effect. The skin effect shifts current toward more superficial layers, lowering resistance and reducing the likelihood of deep thermal injury — an important consideration in clinical use.

Tissues rich in water and ions (for example, muscle and blood) conduct current well. In contrast, dense structures such as bone and relatively hydrophobic or poorly hydrated tissues (adipose tissue and the *stratum corneum*) conduct less efficiently.

2.2.2. Thermal effects of electric current

The amount of heat produced during electrical exposure depends on both the properties of the tissue and the characteristics of the applied current. Importantly, tissues warm up in fundamentally different ways under direct current versus alternating current at low or high frequencies.

Direct and low-frequency currents

Here, heating is driven mainly by **Joule (resistive) heating** — the conversion of electrical energy into thermal energy as current passes through a resistive medium. Because tissues oppose the movement of charged particles, collisions occur, releasing energy as heat.

In biological tissues, the charge carriers are predominantly electrolyte ions (formed when salts, acids, and bases dissociate in water). Typical examples include sodium (Na^{+}), potassium (K^{+}), calcium (Ca^{2+}), and chloride (Cl^{-}). As these ions move and collide within the conductive pathways, their energy is dissipated as heat. The most significant temperature rise occurs along the current path and diminishes with distance from it. At higher intensities, this heating can be intense and challenging to regulate, increasing the likelihood of burns.

High-frequency currents

With high-frequency exposure, the dominant mechanism is **dielectric heating**, resulting from the polarization of water and other polar molecules (dipoles) in the tissue. Key dipolar components in tissues include water, proteins (via polar groups in specific amino acids), phospholipids and ceramides (with polar head groups essential for membrane structure), and nucleotides (which contain asymmetrically distributed polar regions that create dipole moments). In a high-frequency alternating field, these dipoles rapidly reorient, producing microscopic, localized heat generation. This mechanism allows better control over both heating intensity and adequate depth.

High-frequency current also produces so-called **skin effect**, in which the current density shifts toward the surface. This reduces energy deposition deeper in the tissue, helping lower the risk of severe thermal injury and burns.

High-frequency alternating current tends to deliver **more predictable, localized heating** than direct or low-frequency currents, which is why high-frequency approaches are widely used in surgery, physiotherapy, cosmetic dermatology, and other fields where precise thermal targeting and safety are critical.

2.2.3. Non-thermal effects of electric current

Electric current can affect living tissues in ways that are not primarily linked to heating. Key non-thermal effects include:

- **Electrical stimulation of nerves and muscles.** Electric current can activate nerve fibers and muscle tissue by increasing the excitability of electrically responsive cells and supporting the propagation of nerve signals. This principle underlies neuromuscular electrical stimulation (see Part II, section 2.6).
- **Polarization of cell membranes.** As current passes through tissue, charges redistribute within cells and across their membranes. This shifts membrane potential and can influence physiological activity, including metabolism, transport processes, and ion-channel function.

- **Electroosmosis**. An electric field can drive the movement of fluid and ions within tissues. Clinically, this is used to support blood flow, enhance metabolic activity, and improve the delivery of pharmacologically active substances.

These mechanisms are applied across medicine — from physiotherapy and rehabilitation to diagnostic assessment of nerve and muscle function.

In aesthetic body-contouring programs, direct, low-frequency, and pulsed currents are used to act on electrically excitable tissues (e.g., **electromyostimulation** and **microcurrent therapy**) and to facilitate transdermal delivery of active substances (**ionophoresis**).

2.3. Electrotherapy technologies: variants and effects

Electrotherapy approaches can be grouped by the manner in which current is produced within tissues. Three broad categories are commonly distinguished:

1. Resistive
2. Capacitive
3. Inductive

2.3.1. Resistive technologies

In resistive approaches, the skin is in contact with **two or more electrodes**. When voltage is applied, current travels through the tissues located between the electrodes, making the skin an essential part of the circuit. Most electrotherapy systems operate on this principle.

Based on the number and configuration of electrodes, resistive systems are typically described as:

- Monopolar
- Bipolar
- Multipolar

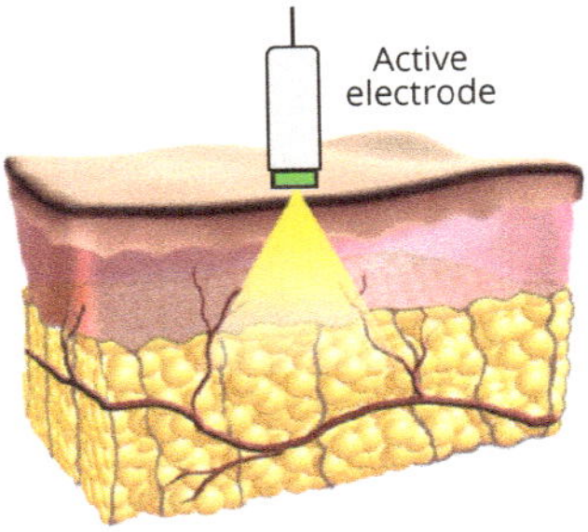

- The active electrode has a relatively small contact area
- The passive electrode has a larger contact area and is positioned at a distance
- The electrodes are not integrated into a single handpiece
- Heating is most intense directly beneath the active electrode and is concentrated in the superficial layers

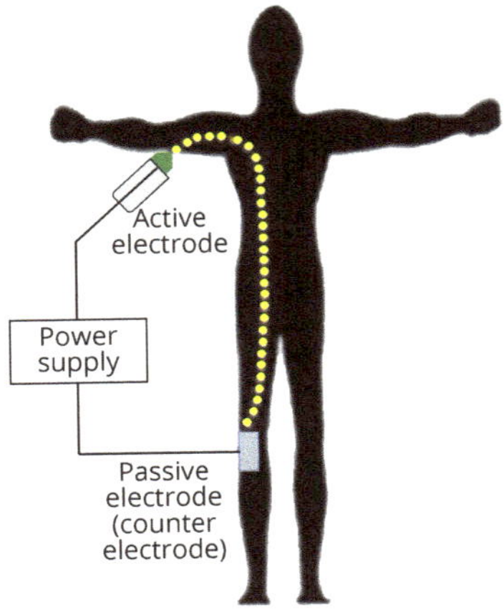

Fig. IV-2-4. Monopolar devices

Monopolar devices

Monopolar systems use two electrodes that differ in size and geometry. A small-surface active electrode is applied to the target zone and moved throughout the session, while a larger passive electrode is placed at a distance and remains stationary (**Fig. IV-2-4**).

With high-frequency alternating voltage, current density is greatest beneath the active electrode and progressively decreases with distance. As a result, the strongest heating occurs at the skin–electrode interface. Because the *stratum corneum* has high resistance, peak temperatures develop there. Reaching therapeutic temperatures in deeper layers, therefore, requires substantial heating of the epidermis, which increases the risk of superficial burns. Given these depth limitations and safety concerns, monopolar RF devices that rely on surface electrodes for thermal skin treatment are used less often and are not appropriate for work with SAT.

Beyond thermal applications, monopolar configurations are used in **electrolipolysis** (see Part IV, section 2.5), **electromyostimulation** (see Part IV, section 2.6.4), and **microcurrent therapy** (see Part IV, section 2.7).

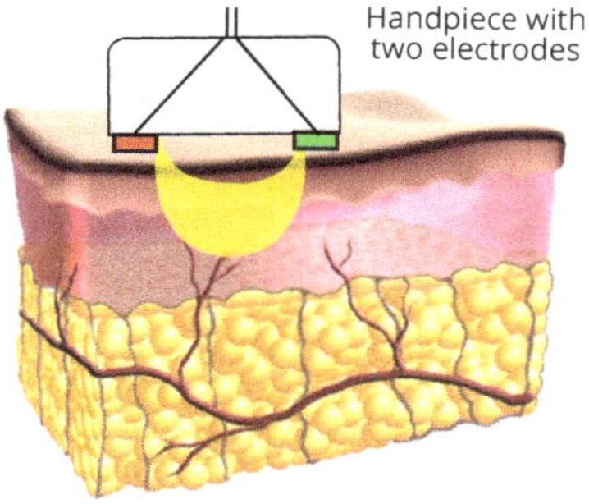

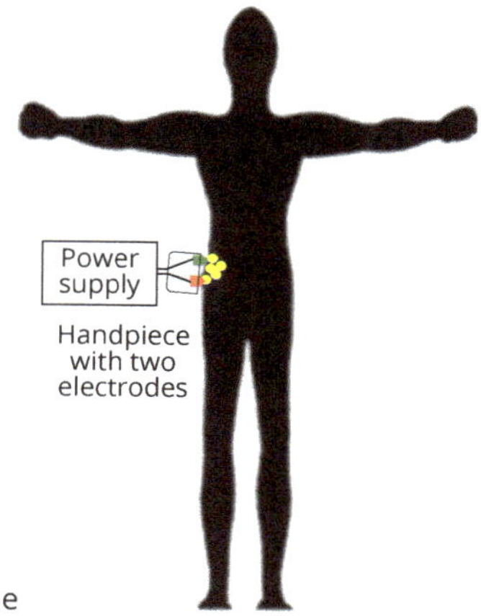

- Two equivalent active electrodes are built into one handpiece
- The electrodes are similar in size and shape
- They are placed close together
- Heating is focused in the tissue volume between the electrodes

Fig. IV-2-5. Bipolar devices

Bipolar devices

Bipolar RF systems employ two closely spaced electrodes, which help confine the treatment zone, improve control over the depth of maximal heating, and reduce the likelihood of superficial burns. Both electrodes are housed in a single handpiece, ensuring consistent skin contact and a fixed distance between them. When a voltage is applied, current flows between the electrodes within a relatively small volume (**Fig. IV-2-5**).

Each electrode produces a similar volumetric heating zone; these zones may overlap, with higher temperatures where they overlap. The depth of the hottest region is typically about half the distance between same-shaped electrodes, though electrode geometry can shift this relationship. Driving the focal zone deeper generally requires higher current intensity to expand the heated volumes and increase overlap — an approach that also raises burn risk. For this reason, non-invasive bipolar RF device is not suitable for adipose-tissue treatment and is mainly used at the dermal level for tightening and lifting (**RF lifting**).

This category also includes **radiofrequency-assisted liposuction (RFAL)**, a widely used minimally invasive surgical technique (see Part IV, section 2.4.1).

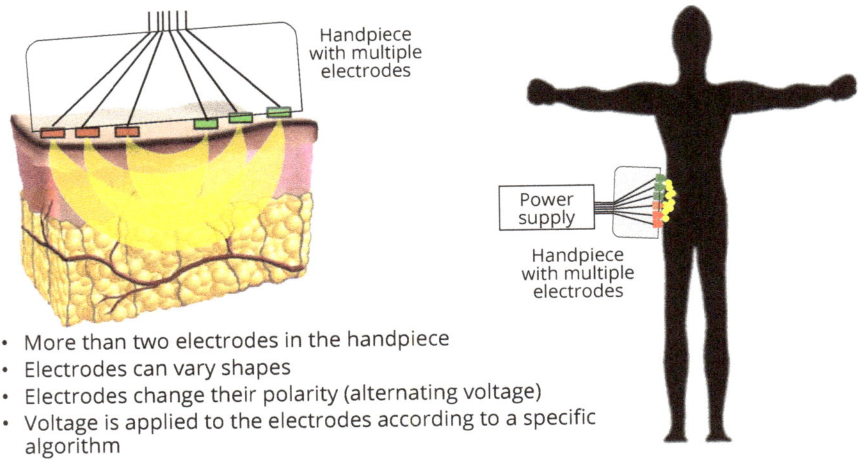

Fig. IV-2-6. Multipolar devices

Multipolar devices

Multipolar systems incorporate multiple active electrodes within a single handpiece. The number, shape, and layout of electrodes vary, and a programmed sequence controls the delivery of voltage. This allows more nuanced management of heating at different depths and markedly reduces the risk of superficial burns (**Fig. IV-2-6**).

Most contemporary non-invasive RF-lifting platforms are multipolar. RF microneedling systems — shown to be effective in anti-cellulite protocols — also belong to this group.

2.3.2. Capacitive technologies

Capacitive approaches differ from resistive ones in that they use two or more insulated electrodes that do not establish direct electrical contact with the skin. The insulating layer (commonly glass, plastic, or ceramic) enables an alternating electric field — sometimes referred to as a "capacitor field" — to couple energy into the body through the insulating surface. Within this field, cations and anions shift in opposite directions. In a steady field, the charge redistribution eventually compensates for the field, and current ceases. In an alternating field, the direction of particle motion reverses with the field, so current continues to flow, producing heating in the medium it traverses.

Capacitive electrodes tend to deliver more substantial, deeper warming, and they preferentially heat tissues with lower conductivity and relatively low water content, such as the *stratum corneum* and SAT.

Example: condenser-type ultra-high frequency (UHF) technologies (**UHF therapy**) (see Part IV, section 2.4.2).

2.3.3. Inductive technologies

In inductive systems, energy is delivered through induction coils (often described as a "coil field") that create a high-frequency alternating magnetic field, rather than through electrodes as in resistive and capacitive approaches. Strictly speaking, there are no electrodes, even though the handpiece may sometimes be labeled an "electrode" because it looks similar externally. When an alternating magnetic field acts on tissues with high electrical conductivity, it induces eddy currents — also known as Foucault currents. Heating develops primarily in water-rich tissues, especially muscle. Because the currents arise within the tissue itself, warming occurs "from the inside," typically increasing temperature by about 2–5 °C at depths of roughly 8–12 cm. In inductothermia, the main therapeutic factor is the internally generated heat, which tends to have a much stronger effect than externally applied heat.

Example: UHF "coil" technology (**UHF inductothermia**) (see Part IV, section 2.4.2).

Alternative current frequency ≠ Pulse frequency

When discussing electric current, the word "frequency" can refer to either how often the current reverses direction (alternating current) or to how it is delivered over time (pulsed mode). For instance, "pulsed (10 Hz, 50 μs) alternating (50 kHz) current" means a 50 kHz alternating current that is delivered as 50 μs pulses repeated at 10 Hz (10 pulses per second). For simplicity, the pulse mode is mentioned only when pulses are actually used.

Expressions such as "low-frequency current" or "high-frequency current" refer to the rate at which the current changes direction. The same logic applies to alternating electric and magnetic fields: they may be delivered continuously or in a pulsed mode.

2.4. High-frequency therapy

High-frequency therapy is an umbrella term for treatment approaches in which a high-frequency electric current is the primary active factor. Different systems can generate these currents in tissue, and they vary in both construction and underlying operating principles.

Most commonly, high-frequency methods rely on resistive coupling — electrodes must be in contact with the skin (**RF therapy**). Other approaches use inductive or capacitive coupling: an UHF electromagnetic field (around 20 MHz) can act without direct contact and induce Foucault (eddy) currents in the skin (**UHF therapy**).

2.4.1. Radiofrequency therapy (RF therapy)

RF therapy delivers alternating current into soft tissues at frequencies up to 6 MHz. These values fall within the broader frequency region associated with radio communications (the high-frequency band, 3–30 MHz). For that reason, the current used in these procedures is commonly referred to as a radiofrequency (high-frequency) current — even though electric current and electromagnetic radiation are not the same phenomenon.

In high-frequency current technologies, **temperature rise is the principal active component**. These methods can be used at both the dermal level and within SAT.

Adipose tissue is electrically non-uniform. Adipocytes, which contain large amounts of hydrophobic lipid, conduct poorly. In contrast, the fibrous septa that partition fat lobules conduct more readily because they contain water associated with proteins. As RF energy heats these septa, the heat then spreads to adjacent adipocytes.

Adipose tissue is temperature-responsive. Warming initiates physiological and biochemical changes in adipocytes that favor lipolysis and suppress lipogenesis (Franco W. et al., 2010). Clinical outcomes depend largely on both temperature and exposure time. At approximately 38–39 °C, fibroblast activity increases, but this range is generally insufficient to trigger meaningful lipolysis. Heating to 43–45 °C and maintaining it for at least 10 min can cause irreversible adipocyte injury and trigger apoptosis. Temperatures above 45 °C may lead to necrosis.

A key benefit of RF-based approaches for cellulite and localized fat is their action on the fibrous septa of SAT: heating promotes fibroblast activity and collagen remodeling. Thickening septa while reducing superficial fat volume lowers the mechanical pressure of fat lobules on the dermis, making surface irregularities less pronounced. At the same time, strengthening the dermal collagen network helps prevent — or substantially reduce — skin laxity in areas where fat volume has decreased (Royo de la Torre J. et al., 2011).

RF current–based techniques used in anti-cellulite and localized fat protocols include:

- RF liposuction
- RF lipolysis
- RF diathermy and electroporation of adipose tissue
- RF microneedling

Radiofrequency current ≠ Radio waves!

The alternating current operating in the RF range (4–5 MHz) is often referred to as "radiofrequency current," and the electrotherapy technique using it is known as "radiofrequency therapy." This terminology arises from a common misconception about the difference between currents of charged particles and electromagnetic waves.

Frequency measures how often an event occurs within a set period. For alternating current, it indicates how often the current changes direction per second. In contrast, for electromagnetic waves, frequency refers to the number of oscillations of the electric and magnetic fields that make up the wave.

Simply because the frequency values for alternating electric current and electromagnetic radiation may match numerically does not mean these two different physical phenomena are identical.

It's crucial to use accurate terminology: "radiofrequency current" and "radiofrequency therapy." Radio waves and their related phenomena are distinct from these electrical concepts.

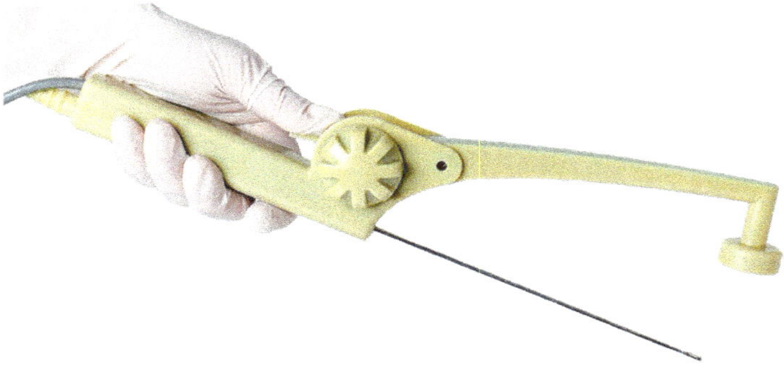

Fig. IV-2-7. RFAL handpiece: minimally invasive bipolar RF technology with aspiration for SAT removal (BodyTite, Invasix, Israel)

RF-assisted liposuction

RFAL is a minimally invasive surgical technique widely considered the current "gold standard" for treating localized fat deposits. It is commonly performed either instead of traditional suction-assisted liposuction or alongside it to improve overall results (Duncan D.I., 2022).

The method was developed and patented by Invasix (Israel), which launched the first commercial system, BodyTite, in 2009 (**Fig. IV-2-7**). The technique uses a bipolar configuration with two electrodes of different geometry housed in a single handpiece; the spacing between them can be adjusted using a dedicated lever. The internal electrode is a cannula introduced into the SAT through a pre-made entry channel. Along most of its length, it is insulated with silicone, leaving only a small exposed segment near the tip. A flat external electrode is placed on the skin directly above the cannula tip. As the cannula is advanced and repositioned within SAT, the external electrode is moved across the skin in parallel, tracking the cannula's path in the same plane. When voltage is applied, current travels between the external electrode and the exposed tip, producing targeted tissue heating (**Fig. IV-2-8**).

Peak temperatures — reported to reach up to about 70 °C — occur in the immediate vicinity of the cannula tip. In this zone, fat is liquefied, vessels are coagulated, and fibrous septa undergo thermal coagulation; the emulsified material is then removed through the cannula by aspiration. Temperature control is supported by multiple sensors built into the electrodes.

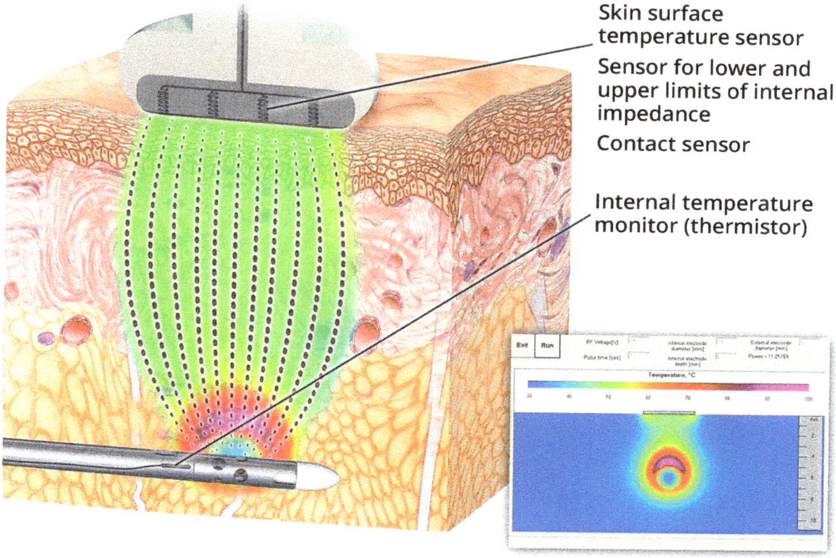

Fig. IV-2-8. Tissue heating profile and temperature control with thermosensors (BodyTite, Invasix, Israel)

After BodyTite, additional handpieces (FaceTite, NeckTite, and AccuTite) were developed for different anatomical areas. They vary in electrode dimensions and heating profiles, but follow the same operating concept. AccuTite, the smallest option, is intended for precision work in delicate regions, including the periorbital area.

Compared with conventional surgical liposuction, this approach also delivers heat to the dermis, which promotes skin tightening and contraction in the treated area. Because heating and aspiration occur simultaneously, the procedure is typically efficient (excluding preparation and local anesthesia). It is also minimally invasive: the small entry sites for the internal cannula usually heal quickly and leave little to no visible scarring.

RF-assisted lipolysis

In contrast to RFAL — where fat is liquefied and physically removed — non-invasive RF lipolysis relies on a gradual, physiologic breakdown of fat that can continue after the session. The temperature rise triggers enzymes that cleave neutral fats (triglycerides) into glycerol and fatty acids. This approach raises two practical issues:

1. Can the SAT be heated to the required range without overheating the layers above it?
2. How can the byproducts of lipolysis be cleared from SAT to reduce the chance of re-uptake by adipocytes?

Commercial solutions address these questions in different ways. For example, ReGen TriLipo Maximus (Pollogen, Israel) combines RF treatment with electromyostimulation. It uses a multipolar handpiece with three or five identical electrodes. A high-frequency alternating voltage is delivered to the electrodes as low-frequency pulses in a programmed sequence. The resulting RF current warms the dermis; heat then propagates into SAT, where it promotes lipolysis. At the same time, electrical impulses trigger contractions in nearby muscles, which may accelerate fatty acid utilization and support microcirculation in the treated area.

Another option is Evolve TRIM technology (Invasix, Israel) (**Fig. IV-2-9**). Six dome-shaped bipolar handpieces are positioned over the target zone. Built-in temperature sensors regulate exposure settings. The handpieces are connected to a vacuum source that generates negative pressure; when the skin is lifted, SAT is drawn between

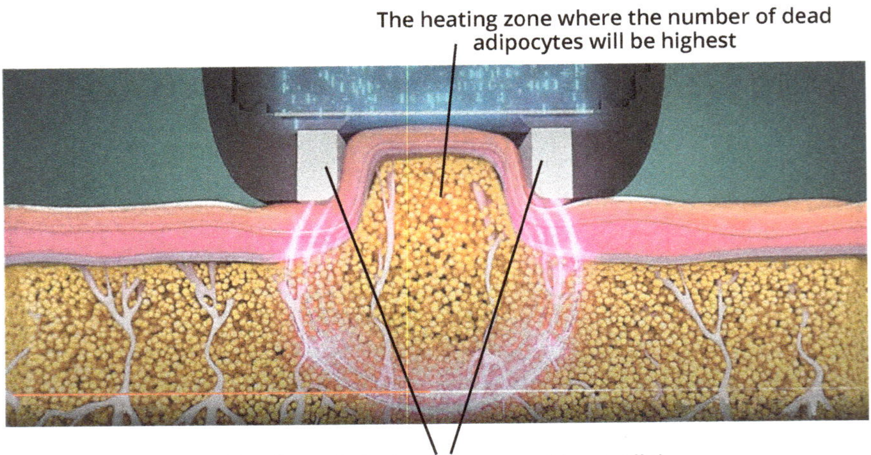

Fig. IV-2-9. Evolve TRIM handpiece (Invasix, Israel): principle of operation

two laterally oriented electrodes. A high-frequency voltage is then applied, driving current into the tissue and producing heat. In this configuration, the region of maximal heating is concentrated in the SAT captured between the electrodes.

RF lipolysis tends to be most effective when used as part of a broader anti-cellulite plan that includes lymphatic drainage massage (to facilitate removal of free fatty acids from adipose tissue) and physical activity (to increase fat "burning").

RF diathermy and electroporation

This non-invasive approach combines RF diathermy with electroporation (Invasix, Israel). Treatment is performed with a multipolar BodyFX handpiece (**Fig. IV-2-10**).

The handpiece has a dome-shaped design and is connected to a vacuum pump. After it is placed on the skin, dermal tissue is drawn into the treatment chamber. High-frequency voltage is then applied, producing RF current flow and heating the tissue to approximately 42–43 °C.

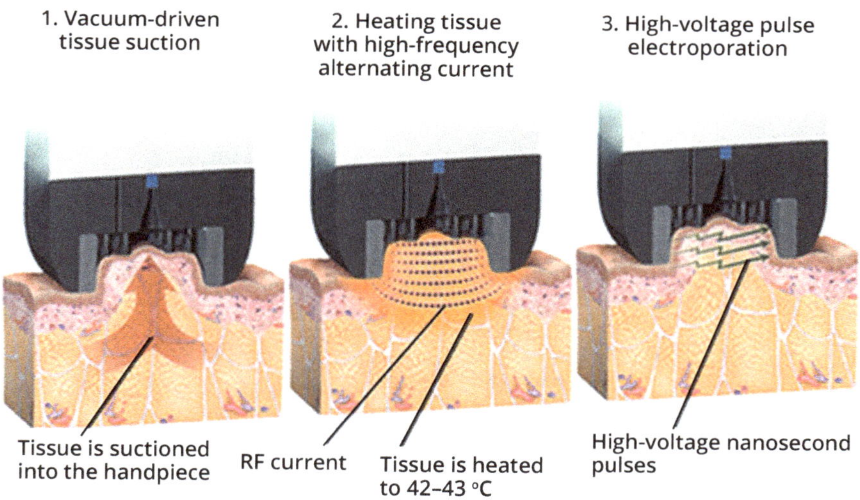

Principle of operation of the BodyFX handpiece (Invasix, Israel):

1. Mechanical disruption initiates tissue regeneration.
2. Focused thermal coagulation prevents bleeding and initiates remodeling.
3. Volumetric heating improves cellular and tissue metabolism.

Fig. IV-2-10. BodyFX handpiece (Invasix, Israel): тon-invasive RF diathermy and electroporation of SAT

Next, very short high-voltage pulses (around 2 kV, < 1 ns) are delivered to induce electroporation of adipocyte membranes. During treatment, a portion of adipocytes and vertical fibrous partitions are irreversibly damaged, while fibroblasts are thermally stimulated. In the following period, affected adipocytes undergo apoptosis, and fibroblasts begin synthesizing new structural proteins as tissue architecture is remodeled. Over time, the skin typically appears smoother and firmer.

A standard anti-cellulite course is often described as consisting of 8 weekly sessions.

RF microneedling

This minimally invasive, multipolar method combines mechanical microneedling (creating multiple microchannels in the skin) with RF energy and is widely regarded as a leading option for tissue remodeling. Many major manufacturers offer their own platforms. Well-known examples include Morpheus8 (Invasix, Israel), MATRIX RF Microneedling (Candela Medical, USA), Infini (Lutronic, South Korea/USA), Scarlet S (Viol, South Korea), among others.

RF microneedling handpieces vary by needle count, arrangement, and insertion depth (**Fig. IV-2-11**). Needle electrodes may be non-insulated or partially insulated, with coating along the shaft and an exposed tip. Voltage-delivery algorithms also differ across systems. Together, these design choices shape the local temperature distribution in the treatment zone and allow clinicians to select configurations suited to different depths and anatomical areas, including the subdermal layer.

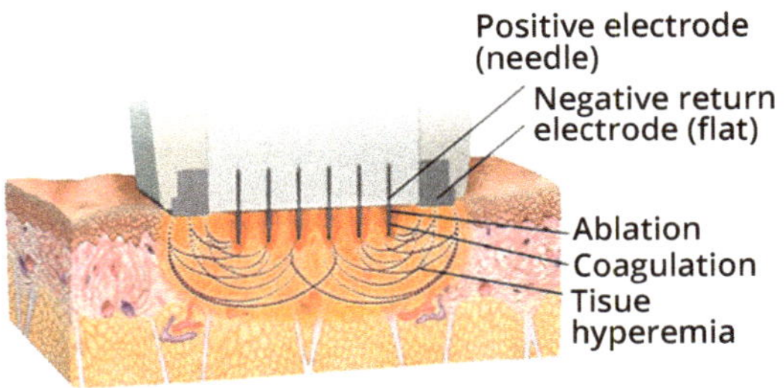

Variable elements in the design of RF handpiece:

1. Number of needle electrodes
2. Shape and contact area of flat electrodes
3. Relative positioning of electrodes
4. Length of needle electrodes
5. Main material of the needles
6. Presence of insulation coating on the needle
7. Total working area of the handpiece

Variable parameters of the energy delivery mode:

1. Power
2. Pulse duration and frequency

Fig. IV-2-11. RF microneedling handpiece (Morpheus8 / Invasix, Israel)

The remodeling response is typically explained by three complementary mechanisms (**Fig. IV-2-12**):

1. Controlled mechanical injury and thermal ablation initiate regeneration.
2. Focal thermal coagulation supports hemostasis.
3. Bulk tissue heating enhances cellular metabolism and activates biochemical repair pathways.

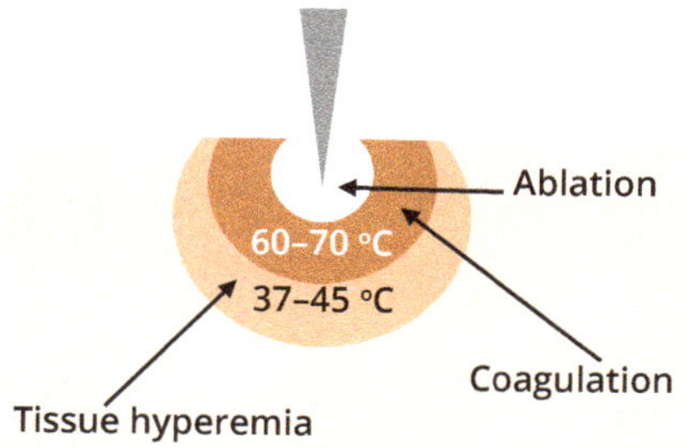

Fig. IV-2-12. Thermal zones

Classic indications include dermal aging and texture concerns — such as skin laxity, wrinkles, enlarged pores, scars, and striae. In anti-cellulite protocols, RF microneedling is often used after surgical liposuction or minimally invasive RFAL to tighten and improve skin quality. Handpieces with 7–8 mm needles can also be used to target localized fat deposits as a standalone approach.

2.4.2. Ultra-high frequency therapy (UHF therapy)

As with RF therapy, the main active factor in UHF therapy is an alternating current that produces tissue heating. The similarity ends there because UHF therapy relies on different physical principles than resistive RF methods.

UHF systems operate without direct contact by generating an alternating electromagnetic field with an oscillation frequency several tens of times higher than the alternating-voltage frequency used in RF technologies (in the MHz range). Common operating frequencies include:

- 27.12 MHz — typical for systems produced in Western markets
- 40.68 MHz — typical for systems produced in Russia and CIS

Based on how the alternating electromagnetic field is generated, UHF technology is commonly divided into two categories:

- **Capacitor-based:** two capacitor plates connected to a UHF field generator create an electromagnetic field (**Fig. IV-2-13**) that primarily affects tissues with low electrical conductivity. The air gap between the plates and the skin influences both intensity and adequate depth: increasing the gap reduces intensity but can allow deeper penetration.
- **Coil-based (magnetic):** the handpiece contains an induction coil (**Fig. IV-2-14**). When activated, a field forms around the coil, inducing eddy currents in tissues of higher conductivity.

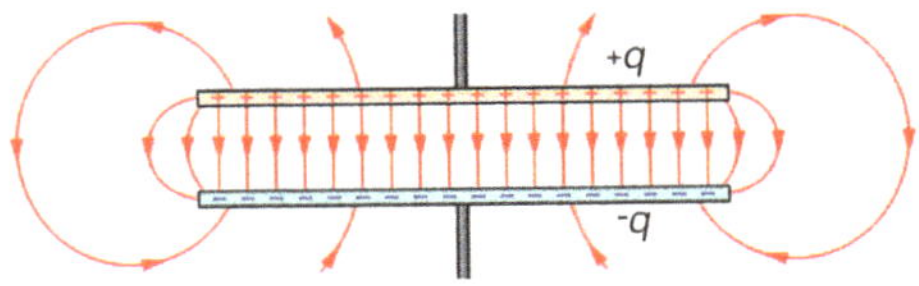

Fig. IV-2-13. Electromagnetic field between the capacitor plates

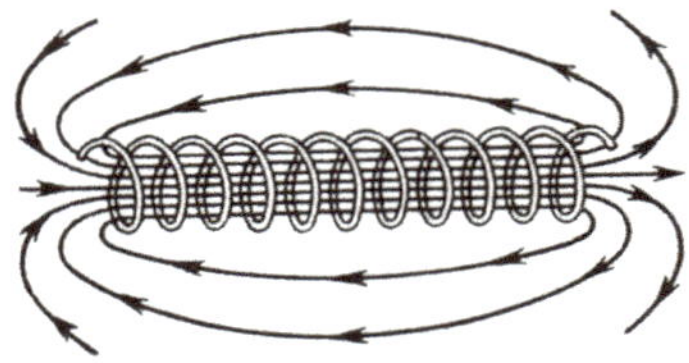

Fig. IV-2-14. Coil electromagnetic field

Propagation of a UHF electromagnetic field is shaped by two sets of factors: the characteristics of the emitter (for example, the geometry, dimensions, and positioning of capacitor plates or inductive coils) and the biophysical properties of the tissues the field passes through.

With capacitor-based systems, the patient is placed between two plates so the field traverses the target region or pathological focus. With coil-based handpieces, the field is delivered directly to the intended zone using a unipolar handpiece.

To distinguish UHF from RF in practical terms: conventional RF technologies act through skin contact and warm deeper layers by driving electric current at roughly 1–6 MHz. UHF technologies, by contrast, work without contact and rely on an alternating electromagnetic field at frequencies above 25 MHz.

UHF therapy effects

An UHF electromagnetic field interacts not only with charge carriers but also with dielectrics — materials that conduct current poorly.

It influences both polar (dipole) and non-polar molecules; in a UHF field, even non-polar molecules can become temporarily polarized, behaving as induced dipoles with partial conductive characteristics. Field strength is greatest near the source and declines with distance.

Because UHF exposure can confer conductive behavior on dielectrics, the effective resistance of biological tissues drops markedly. As a result, the UHF field can penetrate the epidermis, dermis, SAT, and even deeper structures that are less accessible to other energy modalities. Reportedly, the highest energy absorption occurs in the hypodermis (Vecchia P. et al., 2009).

The defining feature of UHF exposure is therefore its ability to heat dielectric-rich tissues directly via molecular motion while reaching relatively deep layers. Since the field reverses direction continuously, both ionic movement and dipole alignment switch direction tens of millions of times per second. This rapid oscillation produces two categories of effects (Mileva K. et al., 2003):

1. **Thermal effects (at high power)**: rapid rotation of dipole molecules generates frictional losses and heat. In parallel, oscillating ions collide with other ions and neutral molecules, with excess energy dissipated as heat.
2. **Non-thermal (oscillatory) effects**: low-intensity fields primarily promote conformational shifts in molecules and modify physicochemical and structural tissue properties. Commonly described oscillatory impacts include:
   - Changes in the colloidal state of the cell cytoplasm
   - Increased protein dispersibility (through disruption of abnormal protein aggregates)
   - Reduced viscosity of the medium
   - Normalization of pH
   - Increased hydration and activity of individual molecules, along with transport systems

Tissue heating leads to increased blood circulation and lymphatic flow, enhanced vascular permeability, reduced vascular tone, stimulation of fibroblast activity, heightened enzyme activity, accelerated metabolism, and modulation of nerve fiber sensitivity. Additionally, changes in tissue pH contribute to increased lymphocyte counts at the site of inflammation and activate phagocytosis, which is actively employed in physiotherapy to treat inflammatory conditions.

In practice, separating thermal from oscillatory effects is difficult because tissue responses reflect their combined action. That said, the intensity and effective depth of responses can be tuned by adjusting technical and procedural settings — most notably output power and, for capacitor-based systems, the distance between the plates and the tissue.

In physiotherapy, practitioners typically use athermal dosing (the lowest available output power) or oligothermal dosing (producing only mild, comfortable warmth). UHF therapy is used for a wide range of indications, including respiratory conditions (e.g., pneumonia, bronchitis), musculoskeletal disorders (e.g., arthritis, arthrosis, radiculitis), injuries (e.g., bruises, sprains, fractures), inflammatory soft-tissue conditions, neuritis and neuralgia, and rehabilitation after surgery or trauma.

In aesthetic practice, higher power settings are used to achieve more pronounced heating. Common applications include:

- Hyperhidrosis therapy
- Fat deposit treatment
- Skin remodeling

UHF technologies

The only **condenser-based UHF platform** specifically used for SAT reduction is BTL Vanquish® ME (BTL Industries, USA), introduced to aesthetic practice in 2013 (**Fig. IV-2-15**). It produces a UHF electromagnetic field at 27.12 MHz and heats SAT to approximately 45–46 °C, while the temperature in the more superficial skin layers typically remains

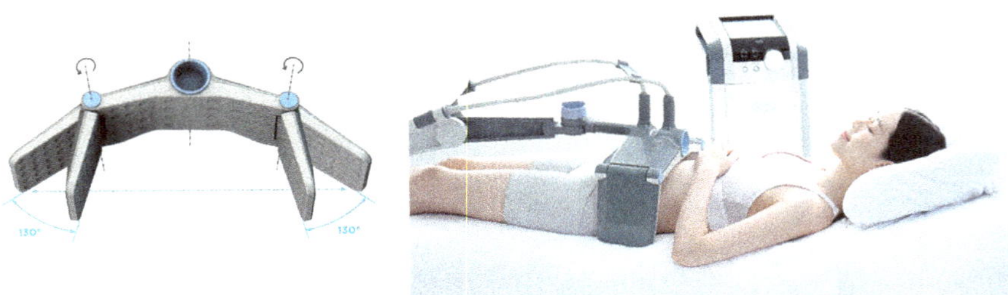

Fig. IV-2-15. BTL Vanquish®ME non-contact UHF lipolysis treatment (BTL Industries, USA)

below 40–41 °C (Kim M. et al., 2017). The handpiece is configured to place the primary heating focus within SAT, so the hypodermis warms more quickly than the skin and underlying muscle. In addition, both the dermis and muscles dissipate heat efficiently via blood flow, whereas fatty tissue cools more slowly. Because the handpiece does not contact the skin, ambient air also helps keep the surface cooler.

Substantial evidence supports the safety and effectiveness of this approach, often referred to as non-contact UHF lipolysis (some sources also use the term non-contact RF lipolysis). Selected examples include the following.

Fajkošová K. et al. (2014) evaluated UHF lipolysis in 40 healthy volunteers (36 women, 4 men) with pronounced subcutaneous fat in the abdomen and waist. Treatments were performed once weekly for 30 min over four sessions. The handpiece was secured using a fixation cup that covered the target area. Power was increased up to 200 W, producing heating of the SAT and the dermis. Abdominal circumference was recorded at baseline and after the final session; photographs and adverse events were documented. Participants also completed self-evaluation questionnaires and rated satisfaction. Tolerability was good; the only reported adverse effect was mild-to-moderate erythema. Thirty-five participants completed the protocol (five withdrew for reasons unrelated to the study). Thirty-two showed a 1–13 cm reduction in abdominal circumference, while three had minimal change (<1 cm). The most plausible explanation for non-response was limited SAT thickness, as the non-responders were the leanest subgroup. Overall, the mean reduction was 4.93 cm and was statistically significant, supporting clinical efficacy.

Long-term durability has also been reported (Fritz K., Salavastru C., 2017). In a follow-up to a prior multicenter prospective study of abdominal SAT excess, participants were re-evaluated 4 years after their last treatment. Biometric data were compared with baseline, and standardized photographs were taken. Thirteen participants were included. In the original study, participants experienced an average waist circumference reduction of 5.88 cm ($P < 0.001$) and a mean weight loss of 1.29 kg. At four years, the same individuals showed a further average waist reduction of 4.42 cm ($P < 0.001$), while mean weight increased by 0.50 kg. In both analyses, waist changes were statistically independent of weight changes ($P < 0.01$). On average, participants maintained about 75.2% of the initial reduction in waist circumference relative to baseline, and none exceeded their baseline circumference. No long-term procedure-related adverse effects were observed. The authors concluded that, with typical weight fluctuations, roughly three-quarters of the maximal waist reduction persisted at four years.

In patients with metabolic syndrome and moderate obesity, UHF-induced lipolysis has been reported to reduce waist circumference significantly. Response appears to correlate with insulin resistance: lower resistance is associated with stronger outcomes (Pumprla J. et al., 2015).

Magnetic resonance imaging (MRI) data also support efficacy. Downie J. and Kaspar M. (2016) studied six participants and measured abdominal SAT thickness by MRI at baseline and again four weeks after treatment. Digital photographs and anthropometric measures (including weight, waist circumference, and skinfold caliper readings) were also collected. Mean fat-layer reduction was 5.36 mm, while body weight remained essentially unchanged.

Coil-based UHF systems are typically used in physiotherapy for mild heating in inflammatory conditions, aiming to improve circulation, reduce inflammation, and relieve pain. In aesthetic medicine, this approach is represented by Polargen (Union Medical, South Korea), which operates at 40.68 MHz. Pilot studies have suggested benefits for non-contact skin tightening and facial contouring (Kim M. et al., 2016; Kim M. et al., 2017), although broad clinical adoption has been limited.

Safety note: UHF procedures require particular caution in patients with metal implants (including dental prostheses) or other metallic foreign bodies, as field exposure in these areas may increase the risk of burns.

2.5. Electrolipolysis

Electrolipolysis is a non-thermal technique that promotes lipolysis using low-intensity electrical currents (pulsed or low-frequency), without relying on tissue heating. Two formats are commonly described (**Fig. IV-2-16**):

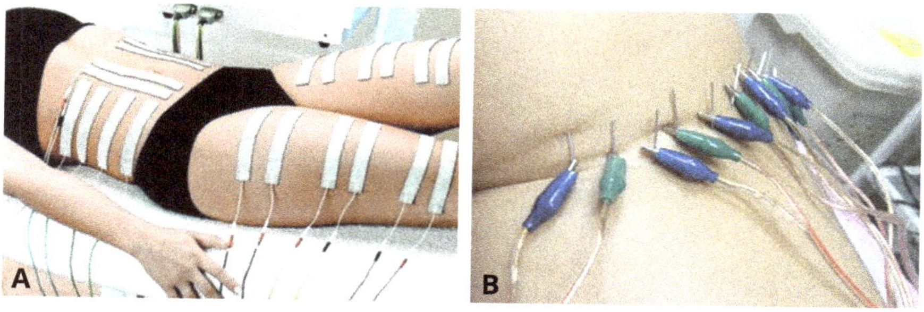

Fig. IV-2-16. Electrolipolysis: A — applicational; B — needle-assisted

- **Non-invasive (surface application):** plate electrodes are placed on the skin, and pulsed currents are delivered.
- **Invasive (needle-assisted):** thin, single-use needle electrodes (typically 8–14) are inserted into the SAT, and low-frequency currents are applied. Needle placement may be barely noticeable for some patients and mildly uncomfortable for others.

Electrical stimulation prompts nerve endings to release catecholamines, which activate lipases that break down triglycerides. Changes in ion distribution near adipocyte membranes can increase membrane permeability. In addition, smooth muscle in vessel walls contracts rhythmically, which can enhance microcirculation in the treated area. Standard target zones include the abdomen, thighs, arms, and buttocks.

A session typically lasts 30–90 min. A standard course is around 10 sessions, usually spaced 5–7 days apart. Combining electrolipolysis with manual lymphatic drainage massage is often recommended to support clearance of metabolic byproducts from SAT.

Overall tolerability is usually good, with minimal discomfort. Patients may feel mild tingling from the impulses, and anesthesia is generally unnecessary. The procedure is relatively straightforward and does not require extensive specialized training. Because the approach is non-invasive, there is typically no downtime, and most people return to normal activities immediately afterward. Transient redness or slight swelling can occur but usually resolves within a few hours.

Some individuals notice early changes after the first session, but the most visible improvement tends to develop progressively as metabolic activity increases. Results are often more apparent after the third or fourth treatment, with peak effects commonly reported 1–2 months after the course is completed.

The method has gained popularity in countries including Thailand, Turkey, Brazil, South Korea, and Mexico, where it is widely offered in aesthetic clinics and beauty centers.

2.6. Neuromuscular stimulation

Modern aesthetic techniques have also emerged that aim to indirectly influence the SAT by activating underlying muscles. The key idea is simple: working muscle needs fuel.

Active muscle requires energy substrates and communicates this demand to the body through signaling molecules called myokines (**Fig. IV-2-17**) (Hoffmann C., Weigert C., 2017). These signals drive adaptive responses across multiple organs and tissues (**Fig. IV-2-18**),

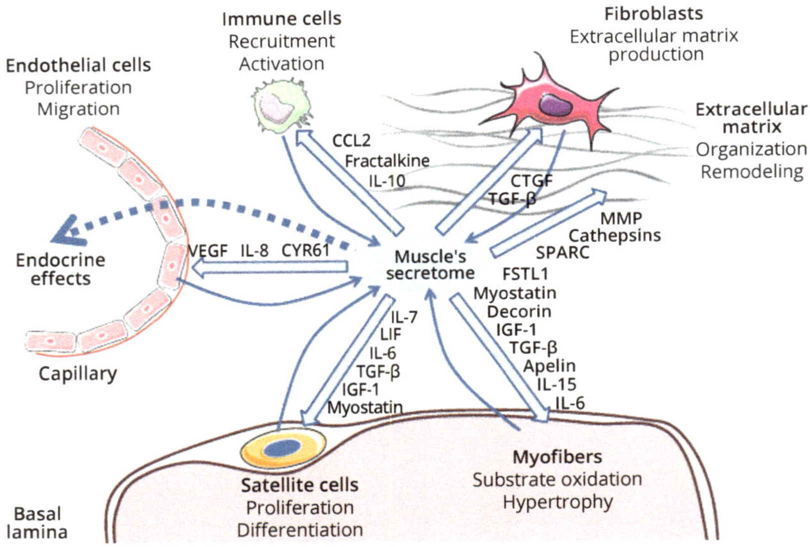

Fig. IV-2-17. Myokines are signaling substances released by muscles (adapted from Hoffmann C., Weigert C., 2017; CC BY)

Abbreviations: IL — interleukin; CCL2 — chemokine (C-C motif) ligand 2; CTGF — connective tissue growth factor; CYR61 — cysteine-rich protein 61; FSTL1 — follistatin-like protein 1; IGF-1 — insulin-like growth factor 1; LIF — leukemia inhibitory factor; MMP — matrix metalloproteinases; TGF-β — transforming growth factor beta; VEGF — vascular endothelial growth factor

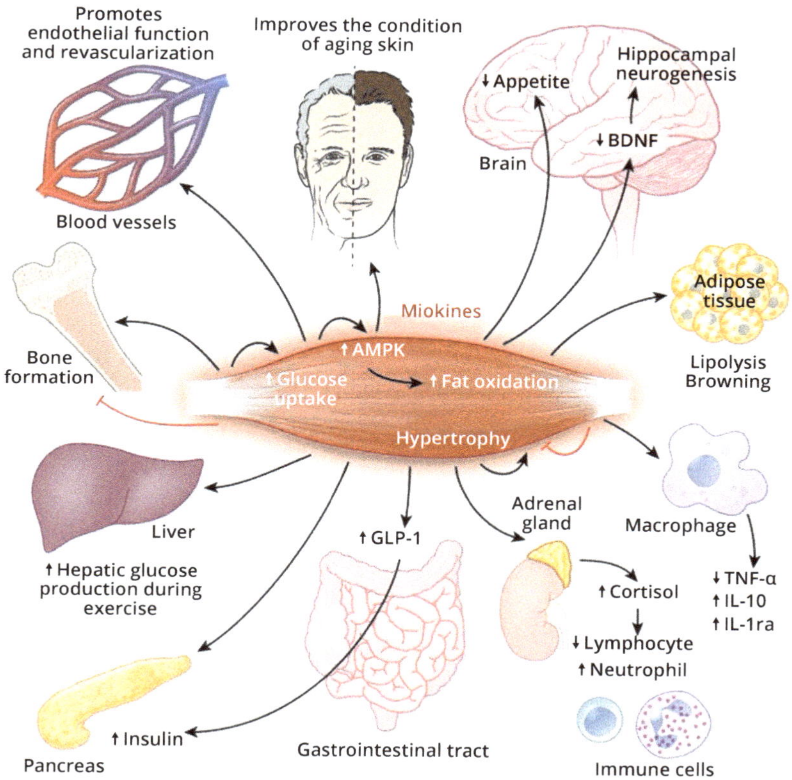

- Myokines are synthesized and released by muscle cells and act through autocrine, paracrine, and endocrine pathways.
- They function as signaling molecules that enable cross-talk between skeletal muscle and other organs.
- The myokine IL-6 is a key mediator of the anti-inflammatory effects associated with physical activity.
- Discovering additional myokines and clarifying their functions could open new directions for drug development.
- Myokines also have potential as biomarkers to monitor response and tailor exercise programs for patients—for example, in diabetes, cancer, and neurodegenerative disorders.

Fig. IV-2-18. Muscles are active participants in hormonal regulation (adapted from Severinsen M.C.K., Pedersen B.K., 2020; CC BY)

Abbreviations: IL — interleukin; CCL2 — chemokine (C-C motif) ligand 2; CTGF — connective tissue growth factor; CYR61 — cysteine-rich protein 61; FSTL1 — follistatin-like protein 1; IGF-1 — insulin-like growth factor 1; LIF — leukemia inhibitory factor; MMP — matrix metalloproteinases; TGF-β — transforming growth factor beta; VEGF — vascular endothelial growth factor

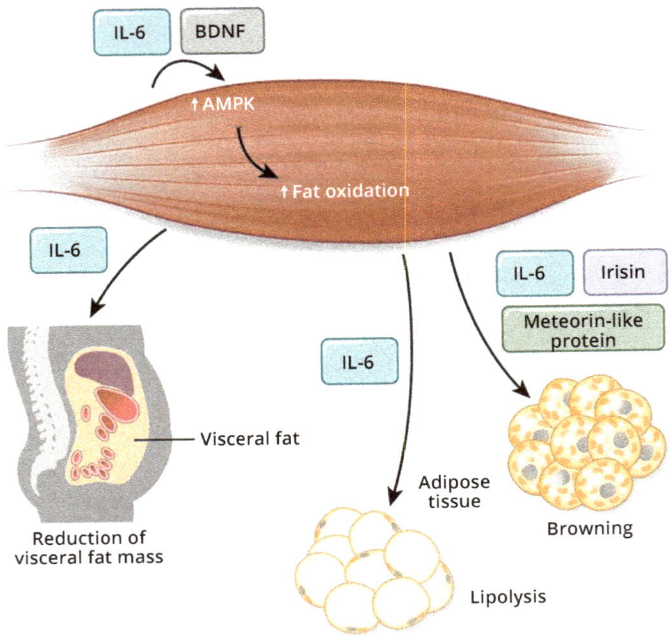

- IL-6 promotes lipolysis and is associated with reduced visceral fat volume.
- Irisin, a meteorin-like protein, and IL-6 contribute to the "browning" of white adipose tissue.
- IL 6 and brain-derived neurotrophic factor (BDNF) enhance AMPK activity — an enzyme central to cellular energy regulation.

Fig. IV-2-19. Muscular activity influences adipose tissue status (adapted from Severinsen M.C.K., Pedersen B.K., 2020; CC BY)

collectively supporting sustained muscle performance (Severinsen M.C.K., Pedersen B.K., 2020). Adipose tissue is a major target because it represents the body's primary reservoir of energy substrates.

Subcutaneous fat stores located closest to the engaged muscle tend to respond first, since the signaling and metabolic "distance" is shortest. When multiple muscle groups are activated intensely, visceral fat may also become responsive to these signals (**Fig. IV-2-19**), which helps explain why consistent, high-intensity training is often associated with gradual reductions in visceral fat.

Muscle activation also increases local blood flow and improves lymphatic drainage. This is critical for delivering oxygen and substrates to the muscle while removing metabolic waste. For adipose tissue, better perfusion and drainage mean faster clearance of lipolysis byproducts from the site where they are produced and a lower likelihood that adipocytes will reabsorb them and re-esterify them into triglycerides (stored fat).

2.6.1. Physiology of neuromuscular stimulation

Skeletal muscle fibers are controlled by motor nerve fibers that arise from large motoneurons in the anterior horns of the spinal cord. After a motor nerve enters the muscle belly, it branches extensively, with each branch supplying anywhere from a few to several hundred muscle fibers. Along each muscle fiber, the nerve terminal forms a specialized contact site — the neuromuscular junction (synapse) — through which the command to contract is delivered.

The sequence is as follows: an action potential travels along the motoneuron's axon toward the periphery. When it reaches the synapse, it triggers the release of a neurotransmitter — acetylcholine — into the synaptic cleft. Acetylcholine then binds to receptors on the muscle fiber's postsynaptic membrane, initiating the cascade that leads to contraction.

If a pulsed electrical current is applied near a nerve ending, it can reproduce the effect of a natural action potential. This provokes acetylcholine release into the synaptic cleft and, in turn, contraction of the muscle fiber. For this response to occur reliably, stimulation settings—especially pulse frequency and intensity — must be selected appropriately. In essence, external stimulation activates the motor pathway that typically initiates voluntary contraction, which is why **neuromuscular stimulation is often described as highly physiological**.

2.6.2. Neuromuscular stimulation technologies: variants and effects

Neuromuscular stimulation is primarily based on pulsed electrical currents. These pulses may be generated by a pulsed electric field or an alternating magnetic field.

Two main technological approaches are used:

1. **Resistive (electric myostimulation):** uses contact electrodes placed on the skin. When voltage is applied, an electric field forms between the electrodes. This was the earliest implementation

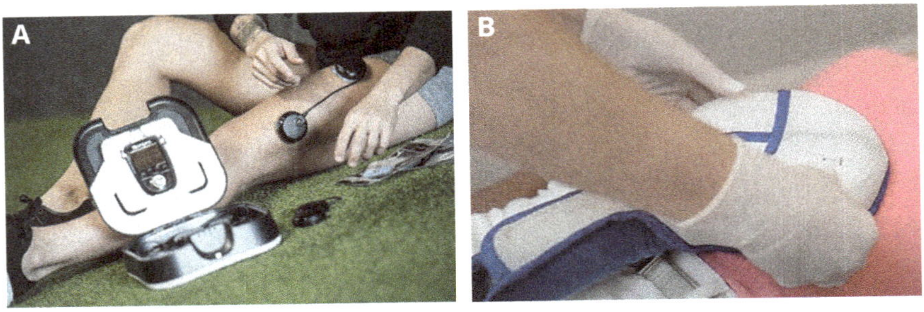

Fig. IV-2-20. Handpieces: A — contact electrodes (electric myostimulation); B — isolated inductance coil (magnetic myostimulation)

and is characterized by two electrodes positioned over or near the target muscle (**Fig. IV-2-20A**).

2. **Inductive (magnetic myostimulation):** uses an induction coil. Alternating current in the coil generates an alternating magnetic field. This approach appeared later; the handpiece is typically flattened and is held at a small distance from the body or placed on the surface with an insulating layer in between (for example, over clothing or a dedicated barrier) (**Fig. IV-2-20B**).

In both cases — whether the primary stimulus is a pulsed electric field or an alternating magnetic field — pulsed electrical currents are induced in tissue and can be detected by nerve endings. Despite this shared endpoint, the two approaches are not interchangeable in practice, because each has distinct operating characteristics that affect how stimulation is delivered and experienced.

Current distribution with depth

With skin-contact electrodes, current density is highest in the superficial layers and steadily attenuates as it travels deeper (**Fig. IV-2-21**). With an inductive coil, the pattern is essentially reversed: induced currents tend to be relatively small near the surface and increase with depth (Weiss R.A., Bernardy J., 2019). As a result, electrode-based stimulation is generally better suited to smaller, more superficial muscles, whereas magnetic stimulation is more effective for recruiting larger, deeper muscle groups.

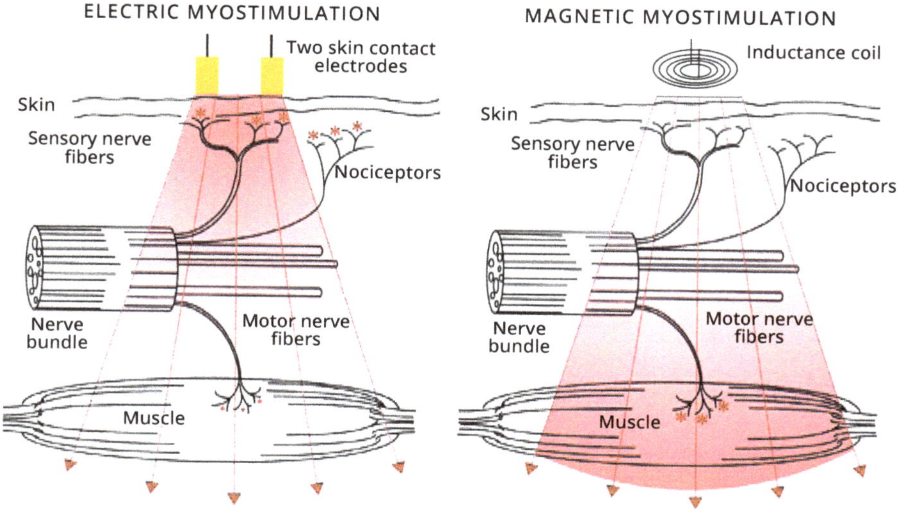

Fig. IV-2-21. Differences in the nerve excitation (red stars) depending on the type of stimulator used (adapted from Weiss R.A., Bernardy J., 2019; CC BY)

Pain and sensory fibers are located closer to the surface, which limits the use of electrical muscle stimulation. The dashed lines schematically show the direction of penetration of the electromagnetic field, while the red shading indicates the intensity of the fields generated by the devices. As shown, magnetic stimulation more selectively affects excitable neuromuscular tissue and allows for greater depth of stimulation.

Subjective sensations during the procedure

Pulsed currents may excite not only motor nerve terminals but also superficial nociceptors. Consequently, electrical stimulation can produce pain that increases as intensity is raised, which effectively limits how far intensity can be escalated to reach deeper musculature.

Magnetic stimulation, in contrast, usually does not cause pain because the induced currents at the level of superficial nociceptors are relatively low and often insufficient to activate superficial muscles. Increasing output can raise superficial induction as well, but it typically amplifies deep muscle contractions even more — something that may feel uncomfortable and may be unnecessary for the clinical goal.

Guidelines for technology selection

When the aim is to "train" superficial, smaller muscle fibers, contact-electrode stimulation is the preferred option. When targeting deeper, larger muscles, magnetic stimulation via an inductive coil is preferred. This feature often makes magnetic approaches especially relevant in sports medicine and rehabilitation, as well as in urology and gynecology. Notably, some systems are chair-based: the patient sits while an alternating magnetic field stimulates the pelvic-floor musculature. A side-by-side comparison of both approaches is provided in **Table IV-2-1** (Vostrikova A.V., 2022).

Table IV-2-1. Neuromuscular stimulation technologies: a comparative table (Vostrikova A.V., 2022)

	ELECTRIC MYOSTIMULATION	MAGNETIC MYOSTIMULATION
Acting factor	Low-intensity direct electric current pulses that mimic the action potential in motor neurons and stimulate the release of acetylcholine	
Handpiece	Two contact electrodes, which are energized in pulse mode	An inductance coil connected to an AC circuit. There is no electrical contact with the skin
How an electric current is generated in the tissue	An electric field is created between electrodes under voltage, in which an electric current begins to flow	An alternating magnetic field that triggers the formation of eddy currents (Foucault currents)
Electric current power with depth	Decreases	Increases
Optimal target	Superficial and smaller muscles	Deep and large muscles, brain
Subjective sensations	Pain may occur (if nociceptors are excited)	No pain, but may be unpleasant with strong muscle contractions

2.6.3. Magnetic myostimulation

A magnetic myostimulation approach for body contouring — High-Intensity Focused Electromagnetic Energy (HIFEM) — was patented by BTL Industries (USA) and introduced commercially in 2018 in the Emsculpt system.

This technology applies a high-power alternating magnetic field to induce electrical impulses in tissue. The result is depolarization of large numbers of motor neurons and synchronous contractions of the muscles within the target zone — reported at roughly 20,000 contractions over 30 min. These contractions are described as supramaximal and cannot be achieved through voluntary exercise.

Supramaximal contractions place exceptionally high demands on the muscle. Adaptation involves structural changes such as increased fiber size and density, culminating in hypertrophy. As workload and hypertrophy increase, muscular energy requirements rise, potentially intensifying lipolysis in nearby fat stores. Triglyceride breakdown may proceed quickly enough that free fatty acids accumulate within adipocytes, triggering programmed cell death (apoptosis). The apoptotic adipocytes are then cleared over subsequent weeks without systemic harm (Gaidash N.V., 2020; Halaas Y., Bernardy J., 2020).

Multiple studies have reported reductions in adipose volume with HIFEM. For example, Weiss R.A. and Bernardy J. (2019) reported evidence of adipocyte apoptosis after a single 30-minute exposure in two Yorkshire pigs, with the apoptotic index increasing from 18.75% to 35.95% at 8 hours. Blood testing showed decreases in triglycerides (51.8%), free fatty acids (28.1%), and glycerol (54.8%), consistent with increased lipid mobilization and utilization. At the same time, creatine phosphokinase rose by 227.8% and lactate dehydrogenase by 35.4%, suggesting an effect on muscle tissue. No adverse changes were observed in skin or adjacent structures. Overall, the findings support a non-thermal pathway for adipocyte loss, accompanied by measurable metabolic effects.

Jacob C.I. and Rank B. (2020) conducted a pilot study on postpartum abdominal contouring in 10 women (3–36 months postpartum; mean age 37.7 years) who received four 30-minute sessions. MRI was performed before treatment and at 1, 3, and 6 months to measure abdominal fat thickness, rectus abdominis thickness, and inter-rectus distance. Weight, standardized photographs, and comfort ratings (1–7 scale) were also collected. MRI showed mean reductions in fat thickness of 17% at 1 month and 20.2% at 3 months; rectus thickness increased by ~20.5% at 1 month and 21.3% at 3 months. Inter-rectus distance decreased by 16.7% at 1 month and 22.7% at 3 months.

At 6 months, the nine remaining participants showed an average 17.6% fat reduction, a 21.7% increase in muscle, and a 23.2% reduction in separation, with relatively stable weight. The authors concluded that HIFEM can reduce subcutaneous fat and rectus separation while strengthening the abdominal wall in postpartum patients, with improvements persisting through follow-up (Jacob C.I., Rank B., 2020).

Since 2020, combined protocols pairing non-thermal HIFEM with thermal RF (heating up to ~40 °C) have been активно studied. Clinical findings across multiple facial and body areas are supported by histology and other laboratory methods.

For instance, Goldberg D.J. (2025) reported that a single non-invasive HIFEM + RF session induced apoptosis in chin fat. During treatment, HIFEM and RF were delivered simultaneously to the target area, affecting skin, adipose tissue, and weakened muscles (the report also references the anterior abdomen and the biceps). In a six-participant group, caspase-7 increased by 511% at 24 hours and by 101% at 7 days, while Bcl-2 decreased by 89% and 24%, respectively; no comparable changes were seen in controls. Post-treatment, adipocytes were smaller and less uniform in shape. Participants generally rated the session as comfortable, and no adverse effects were reported. The authors concluded the method is safe and effective for reducing subcutaneous fat via apoptosis.

In a multicenter study of 34 participants, Jacob C. and Weiss R.A. (2023) evaluated forearm treatment using four 30-minute HIFEM + RF sessions spaced one week apart. MRI at baseline, one month, and three months showed significant reductions in SAT (22.3% at one month; 25.5% at three months), along with increased muscle mass (21.5% at one month; 23.9% at three months). Most participants reported satisfaction (84.64%), high comfort (91.18%), and low pain (mean VAS score 1.58/10).

2.6.4. Electromyostimulation

Electromyostimulation (EMS) uses electrical pulses to elicit muscle contractions. It has been employed for decades in sports medicine — for competition preparation, reduction of muscle soreness, and post-injury recovery — and in rehabilitation medicine to help restore muscle function after trauma or disease. The method is widely regarded as effective and safe, is generally comfortable for patients, and is simple to administer, which aligns well with core requirements for clinical treatments.

In recent years, EMS has also been applied to aesthetic and gynecological concerns associated with altered muscle tone. Among contemporary solutions in aesthetic practice, EVOLVE TRANSFORM technology (InMode, Israel) combines EMS with RF therapy. These modalities complement one another: RF warming of deeper skin layers can increase the responsiveness of subcutaneous fat to myokines that promote lipolysis. Improved microcirculation in the treated region may also support faster transfer and utilization of lipolysis products by nearby muscles. Clinically, this can translate into a visible reduction of localized fat deposits. In addition, RF exposure supports collagen fiber tightening and skin firming in the treated area.

It is worth reiterating that **EMS primarily recruits superficial muscle groups,** and this offers specific advantages (Vostrikova A.V., 2022):

- First, superficial muscles lie close to subcutaneous fat depots, so their increased demand for energy substrates is likely to be met first by SAT.
- Second, activation of superficial muscles enhances microcirculation within the skin and underlying tissues, which generally supports local metabolic processes.

2.7. Microcurrent therapy

Microcurrent therapy is a multimodal technique that uses very low-amplitude, modulated pulsed currents in the microampere range (1 μA = 1/1,000,000 A) with low intensity and adjustable frequency characteristics for therapeutic and cosmetic purposes.

The proposed biological basis of microcurrent therapy involves **modulation of voltage-gated ion channels**. Under microcurrent exposure, sodium and potassium ions redistribute, shifting the membrane potential. This polarity change persists for roughly 1–2 ms in epithelial cells and 3–5 ms in skeletal muscle cells. During this window, divalent cations — especially calcium — enter the cell. Calcium acts as a potent physiological signal and is thought to initiate intracellular cascades that include increased ATP production and greater energy availability for metabolic processes (Cheng N. et al., 1982).

A commonly cited sequence is:

Microcurrents
↓
Change in membrane potential
↓
Opening of ion channels (including calcium channels)
↓
Rapid calcium influx along the concentration gradient
↓
Rise in intracellular calcium
↓
Activation of Ca^{2+}-dependent enzymes
↓
Increase in ATP synthesis (to support downstream metabolism)
↓
Enhanced synthesis of proteins, lipids, DNA, and other key molecules (also aided by increased transport of substrates — amino acids, sugars, etc. — into the cell)
↓
Faster cell differentiation and tissue regeneration

Metabolic activation is considered the central outcome of microcurrent therapy, which helps explain its broad use in cosmetology protocols. At the same time, its effects on muscle tissue are also significant. Because muscle and nerve cells are highly responsive to electrical stimuli, they can be influenced even by tiny currents. In microcurrent therapy, however, current amplitude and pulse duration are kept low—closer to the levels of neuron-generated signals (often described as subthreshold action potentials) — and can be considered relatively physiological.

Unlike EMS, which uses currents in the milliampere range (tens to hundreds of times higher) and produces overt contractions, microcurrent therapy does not cause active muscle contraction. Instead, it is commonly described as helping normalize muscle tone — reducing hypertonus and improving hypotonia.

This gentle influence may provide additional benefits. Subtle alternating tightening and relaxation of muscle fibers under microcurrent exposure can act like a pump: during contraction, small blood and lymphatic capillaries between fibers are compressed; during relaxation, their lumens reopen and refill. The resulting drainage effect can persist for about a day. Unlike manual massage, microcurrent therapy can be used even when the skin is significantly compromised, making it a valuable option for edema management.

In addition, microcurrents affect arteriolar smooth muscle by altering vessel-wall tone. Through this pathway, microcurrent stimulation can improve microcirculation, accelerate the resolution of swelling, and help normalize local metabolism.

2.8. Gel for electrotherapy procedures

During treatments that use **resistive technology,** a conductive **gel must be applied to the skin.** Its primary role is to improve electrical coupling between the metal electrodes and the skin surface. This is important because the *stratum corneum* contains relatively little water (about 15% by weight), which makes it a high-resistance layer. By lowering this barrier, the gel allows current to pass through the *stratum corneum* more efficiently, helps distribute current more evenly, and reduces the likelihood of localized overheating. It also improves electrode-to-skin contact, which can lessen unpleasant sensations such as tingling or pain during the session.

The gel's conductivity is primarily due to water and dissolved electrolyte salts (e.g., sodium or potassium salts). Polymeric thickeners (such as glycerol, carbomer, and polyacrylates) give the gel appropriate viscosity so it stays in place and maintains stable contact. Preservatives are a key component, preventing microbial growth and keeping the product safe throughout its shelf life. Conductive gels do not require added active ingredients, although some formulations may include mild antiseptic components.

Correct application is essential for consistent results. In most cases, a 2–4 mm layer — roughly 15–30 g per treated zone — is sufficient, with the exact amount depending on the area size and the manufacturer's recommendations. The gel should be spread uniformly using a spoon, spatula, or directly from the tube. After the electrode is placed, press it gently to ensure the gel distributes evenly and air pockets are eliminated. If the gel dries out or is removed during the procedure, it can be reapplied to preserve stable, long-duration contact.

For **non-contact UHF procedures** that use capacitive or inductive coupling, **gel is not required**.

Chapter 3
Sound technologies

Sound is a physical phenomenon in which mechanical vibrations travel through a material medium as elastic waves, whether solid, liquid, or gas. Unlike electromagnetic waves, sound cannot propagate in a vacuum; it requires matter (atoms and molecules) to oscillate and pass the vibration along.

In aesthetic practice, sound-based treatments are used for a range of indications, including the management of cellulite and localized fat deposits. Depending on the signal parameters, two main categories are commonly distinguished:

- **Ultrasound therapy** uses ultra-high-frequency (500–3000 kHz) sound waves for therapeutic and preventive purposes.
- **Shockwave therapy** uses low-frequency (16–25 Hz) sound waves, below the range of human hearing.

3.1. Ultrasound therapy

How deep an ultrasound reaches depends largely on frequency: **the higher the frequency, the more superficial the effect.**

- **Low-frequency** (20–45 kHz): ~8–14 cm
- **Medium-frequency** (800–1000 kHz): ~4–6 cm
- **High-frequency** (1600–3000 kHz): ~1–2 cm
- **Ultra-high frequency** (10 MHz): ~0.6 cm

At the SAT level, high-intensity ultrasound can be delivered using different parameter sets and operating modes, which change how it interacts with cells and tissue (Elhelf I.A.S. et al., 2018):

- Low-frequency/high-frequency
- Continuous/pulsed
- Radial/focused

3.1.1 Ultrasonic cavitation (low-frequency ultrasound)

Ultrasonic cavitation is most often associated with **high-intensity, low-frequency** (typically ~37–42 kHz) ultrasound and is primarily a **non-thermal** phenomenon.

When ultrasound passes through a liquid medium, it creates alternating phases of compression and rarefaction (lower pressure). During the rarefaction phase, sufficiently negative pressure can lead to the formation of small voids in the fluid — **cavitation bubbles** (from Latin *cavitas* — void). In practice, these bubbles usually form around pre-existing microscopic gas inclusions, which serve as nuclei for cavitation.

Bubble size depends strongly on frequency: the higher the frequency, the smaller the bubbles. For example, at 20 kHz, cavitation bubbles may reach a radius of about 150 μm, whereas at 3 MHz they are on the order of ~1 μm. As the pressure cycles continue, bubbles can enlarge and coalesce into larger gas cavities (**Fig. IV-3-1**). When

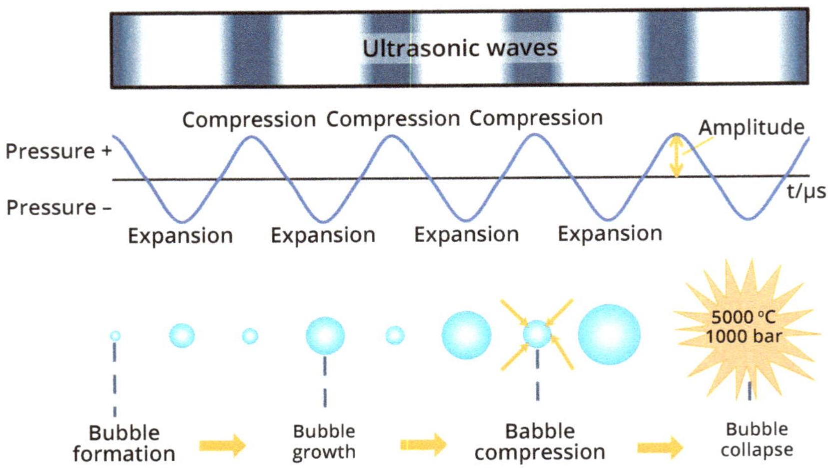

Fig. IV-3-1. Ultrasonic cavitation mechanism: bubbles form, grow, and reach a critical (resonance) size; once that threshold is crossed, they rapidly expand and then collapse ("explode") (adapted from Cao L. et al., 2024; CC BY)

they enter a higher-pressure zone — or during the subsequent compression half-cycle — they may collapse. This collapse generates shockwaves and releases substantial energy.

At the SAT level, this mechanical energy can disrupt the adipocyte envelope, leading to cell death. Cells that are more distended by lipid content tend to be affected first because their membranes are under greater tension. Importantly, ultrasound vibrations used for SAT-level treatment are described as sparing other structures — such as vessels, muscles, and other skin cells — making the effect relatively targeted.

Lipids and cellular debris released after adipocyte injury are taken up by macrophages and cleared from the treated area through lymphatic pathways. Reportedly, this process does not adversely affect the lipid profile or liver function.

Focused vs. non-focused delivery

With **focused ultrasound**, vibrations generated by a specially shaped concave emitter converge in an hourglass-like pattern. The intersection point — the focus — is where ultrasound energy density is highest and where the most substantial effect is produced (**Fig. IV-3-2**). This geometry limits exposure outside the focal zone and supports precise control during treatment. The associated temperature rise in the treatment area (up to 0.9 °C) is minimal. One example of a system based on ultrasonic cavitation is UltraShape (Candela, USA).

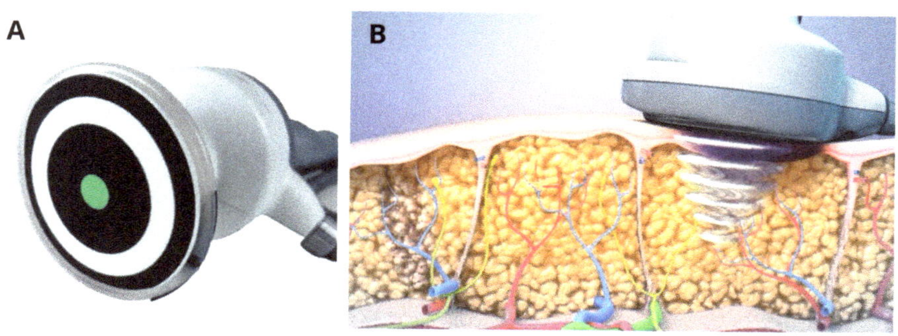

Fig. IV-3-2. UltraShape handpiece (Candela, USA):
A — overall view; B — operating principle
(https://www.youtube.com/watch?v=W4Linv-ebnA)

Non-focused ultrasound can also be used, but it inherently involves greater energy dispersion. One engineering approach aimed at reducing these losses is the UltraWave handpiece for the Accent PrimeX platform (Alma Lasers, Israel). UltraWave uses two main ultrasound modes — longitudinal and transverse — and combines them to target fat cells preferentially. In this configuration, the center of the treatment zone predominantly receives longitudinal waves (associated with skin heating). At the same time, the peripheral region is exposed to transverse (shear) waves, which produce more substantial mechanical effects in tissue.

The handpiece design includes a conical cavity that causes ultrasound waves to diverge on one side and resonate and intensify on the other. Energy is delivered in pulses at 10 Hz, which enhances the mechanical effect via soft shockwaves. A vacuum in the center improves coupling and lifts the skin, positioning SAT more centrally within the ultrasound field (**Fig. IV-3-3**). Together, these features are intended to reduce energy loss and increase effectiveness in SAT treatment while maintaining comfort and minimizing side effects (Verner I., 2021).

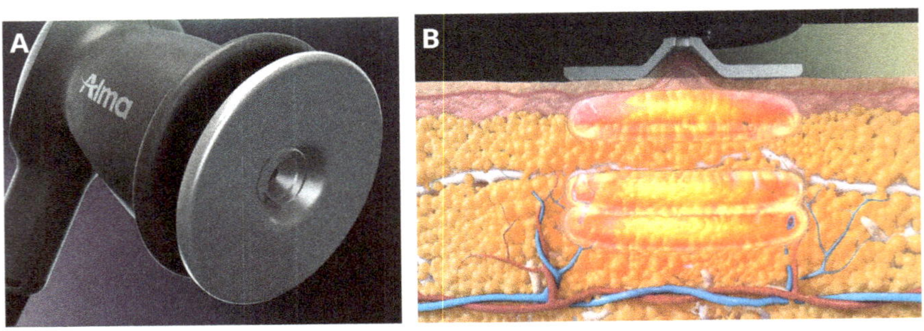

Fig. IV-3-3. UUltraWave handpiece (Accent PrimeX platform, Alma Lasers, Israel): A — overall view; B — operating principle (https://almalasers.com/ tech/ultrawave/)

3.1.2. Ultrasonic thermocoagulation (high-frequency ultrasound)

In contrast to low-frequency ultrasound, high-frequency ultrasound (around 2 MHz) produces a meaningful **temperature rise** in tissue, and most of its clinical effects stem from controlled heating. This approach, commonly referred to as high-intensity focused ultrasound (HIFU), can target soft tissues at substantial depths. Clinically, it is used not only for body concerns but also for non-surgical SMAS lifting by treating deeper facial support structures.

When the goal is to affect adipose tissue, ultrasound at roughly 2 MHz may be delivered at intensities around 1000 W/cm^2. The key is focusing on the focal point, where ultrasound energy is efficiently converted into heat. Molecules within the focal zone oscillate rapidly, and friction between them generates thermal energy, warming the soft tissue (**Fig. IV-3-4**). Temperatures at the focus typically reach 58–70 °C, producing coagulative necrosis.

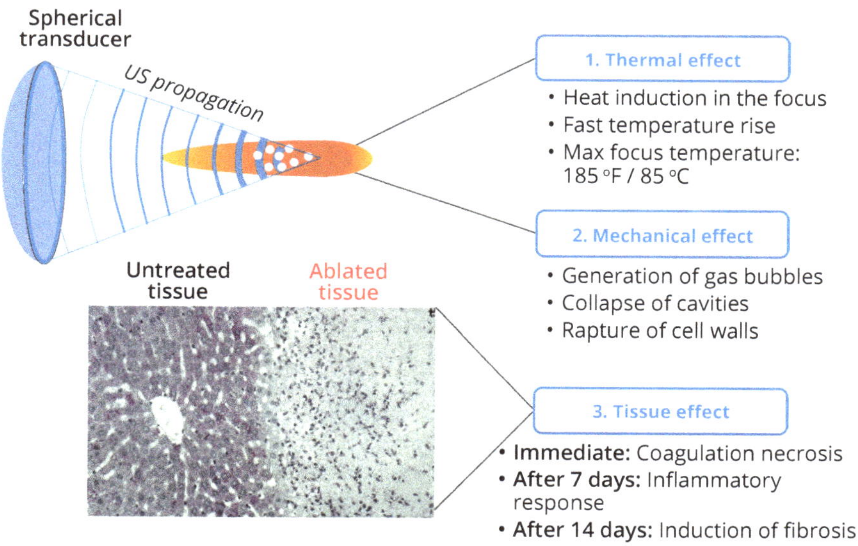

Fig. IV-3-4. Tissue effects of HIFU (https://austinurologyinstitute.com/cancer-care/hifu/)

More than 90% of the total energy is concentrated within the focal zone, which helps protect surrounding tissues outside the thermocoagulation area. That said, cavitation bubbles can still occur; if they collapse, they may contribute to adipocyte injury (see Part IV, section 3.1.1).

The dimensions of each thermocoagulation zone are directly related to delivered power. Each lesion is shaped like an inverted cone. The widest part (upper pole) is typically about 0.5–0.75 mm, and the height ranges from roughly 0.75 to 1.5 mm, depending on the handpiece. Unlike ultrasonic cavitation, high-frequency focused ultrasound also acts on the fibrous septa within the fat layer, promoting their densification, reducing fat lobules, and leading to visible skin tightening.

Macrophages clear cellular debris and liberated lipids, and the treated skin typically heals without complications. Importantly, this process is not accompanied by the inflammatory wound response seen after surgery or lipolytic injections, and it is not associated with systemic disturbances in internal organs or blood parameters (including plasma lipids).

Examples include Ulthera System (Merz, USA), Doublo (Hironic, South Korea), Ultraformer (Classys, South Korea), LipoSonix (Solta Medical, CIF), and others.

A comparison of ultrasonic cavitation and ultrasonic thermocoagulation is provided in **Table IV-3-1**.

Table IV-3-1. Ultrasonic cavitation vs. ultrasonic thermocoagulation

	ULTRASONIC CAVITATION	ULTRASONIC THERMOCOAGULATION
Ultrasound parameters	Low-frequency, high-intensity ultrasound; focused or non-focused	High-frequency, high-intensity focused ultrasound
Main active factor	Cavitation bubbles 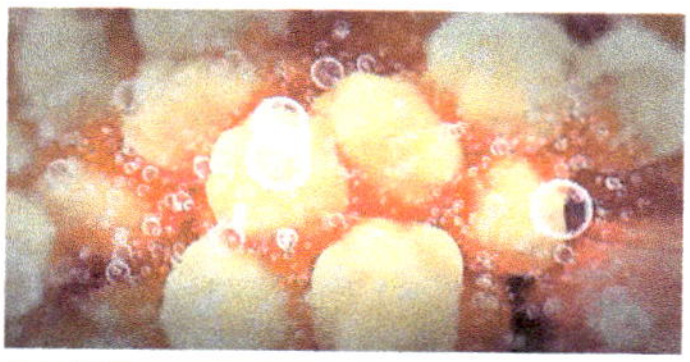	High temperature at the focus 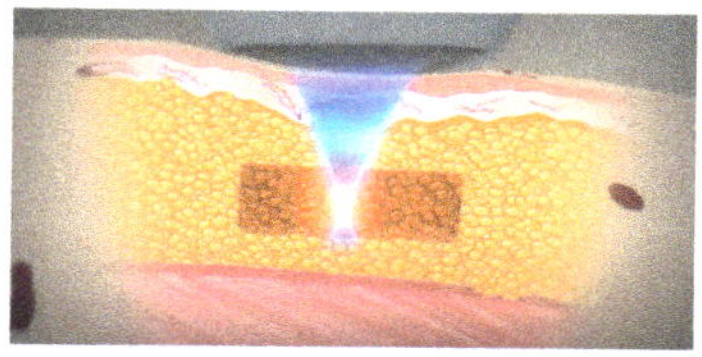
Mechanism of action	Multiple bubbles form within the exposure zone. If bubble collapse occurs close to the cell membrane, the membrane can be irreversibly disrupted, leading to cell death. **The effect is described as selective: adipocytes are affected, while nerves, vessels, and connective-tissue septa are not.**	Tissue is destroyed through rapid heating at the focal point, with temperature rising up to 70 °C within 1–2 s, resulting in coagulative necrosis. **The effect is non-selective within the focal zone: all tissue components in the focus are affected.**
Indications	• Fat folds • Cellulite (any severity) • Sequelae after liposuction or lipolytic injections (residual fat accumulation presenting as lumps)	• Cellulite • Localized fat deposits • Sagging skin
Target areas	• Abdomen • Back • Flanks • Buttocks • Thighs	• Outer and inner thighs • Abdomen • Buttocks • Inner arms
Side effects / tolerability	• Typically painless • Swelling may occur	• Pain • Redness, swelling, mild tingling in the treatment area • Hematomas
Examples	LipoSonix / Solta Medical (USA)	UltraShape / Candela (USA)

3.2. Extracorporeal shockwave therapy

Extracorporeal shockwave therapy delivers acoustic waves in the 16–25 Hz range to the body. Because this is below the threshold of human hearing, these are considered infrasound. The energy is delivered as short, high-pressure pulses that can reach up to 120 MPa.

These pulses are called shockwaves and have several characteristic features: nonlinearity; a pronounced pressure peak followed by a tensile (stretching) component; a speedy rise time; and a short overall duration of about 10 ms (**Fig. IV-3-5**).

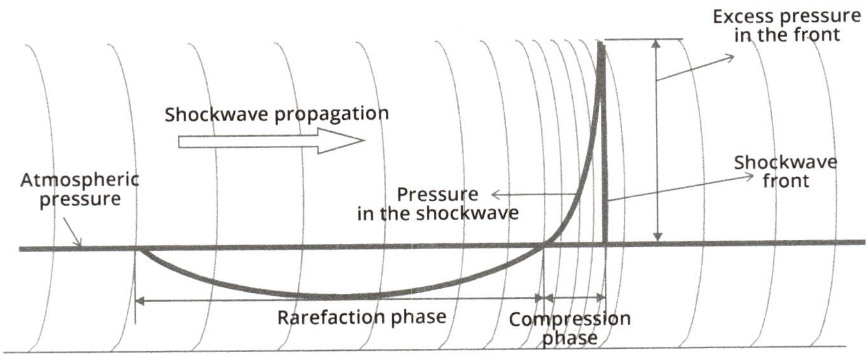

Fig. IV-3-5. Pressure profile during shockwave propagation

A shockwave is a rapidly moving compression front that travels faster than the speed of sound and spreads outward from the source. As the front reaches a given point, pressure rises abruptly to a peak; air density, particle velocity, and temperature increase as well. This is followed by a compression phase during which pressure remains elevated, then returns to atmospheric levels. Next comes an expansion (rarefaction) phase, where pressure drops below atmospheric pressure to a minimum and then gradually returns to baseline. The maximal pressure drop during rarefaction does not exceed 0.3 kg•s/cm^2.

3.2.1. Shockwave effects on SAT

Each shockwave includes two alternating phases — positive and negative — reflecting opposite directions of pressure change. Together, they shape how shockwaves interact with tissue.

1. **Positive phase**: pressure exceeds atmospheric pressure, resulting in firm compression of the tissue. The pressure peak leads to mechanical deformation.
2. **Negative phase**: pressure drops below atmospheric pressure, creating local rarefaction. This environment favors cavitation bubble formation. These gas bubbles may collapse rapidly, releasing energy and producing additional localized mechanical effects — including secondary shockwaves and transient temperature spikes. This contributes to therapeutic outcomes such as disrupting calcifications, improving blood flow, and supporting tissue repair.

Shockwave therapy was first reported for cellulite treatment in 2005 (Siems W. et al., 2005). The authors suggested that even a single self-administered session could improve the appearance of cellulite, associated with a marked reduction in plasma malondialdehyde — a biomarker of oxidative stress.

Several mechanisms may explain the benefits of shockwave therapy for cellulite and localized fat deposits (Modena D.A.O. et al., 2022):

- Micro-injury to the extracellular matrix triggers physiological responses that reshape the extracellular environment, enhance microcirculation, and increase blood and lymph flow.
- Fibroblast activation via mechanotransduction through mechanoreceptors (see Part IV, section 1.1), contributing to remodeling of fibrotic septa in SAT.
- Induction of lipolysis and/or apoptosis in adipocytes.

There are no reports of severe adverse reactions related to shockwave therapy for cellulite treatment (Wigley C.H. et al., 2023). However, patients may experience discomfort from the device noise during the procedure. To reduce this, using ear protection is recommended.

3.2.2. Radial and focused shockwave therapy

Focused and radial shockwave therapy differ in several practical, technically essential ways:

1. How the wave is generated (**Fig. IV-3-6**):
   - **Focused shockwaves** are produced using electromechanical methods (for example, spark discharge, electromagnetic sources, or piezoelectric crystals). These approaches generate acoustic pulses that are then concentrated within tissue using reflectors, creating a point of maximum pressure.
   - **Radial shockwaves** are created when a projectile is accelerated through a guide tube and strikes a metal transmitter at high speed. The impact on the skin surface generates a pressure wave that propagates into the tissue.
2. Focusing precision and energy delivery (**Fig. IV-3-7**):
   - **Focused shockwaves** can be aimed with high accuracy at a chosen point within tissue. However, structures along the propagation path (such as bone or calcifications) can reduce the energy that actually reaches the target. In muscle, for example, energy at the target may drop by more than 50% compared with that in water-based media during propagation.
   - **Radial shockwaves** are less sensitive to "obstacles" along the pathway, so the pulse tends to pass through soft tissue with relatively small energy loss.
3. Depth of impact:
   - **Focused shockwave therapy:** the region of highest energy (the focus) is located deeper — up to 12.5 cm.
   - **Radial shockwave therapy:** the area of highest energy is superficial — near the contact point between the applicator and the skin.

Both approaches are considered adequate for the management of cellulite. A meta-analysis of 11 clinical studies (including 5 randomized controlled trials, 5 cohort studies, and 1 case report) supports the benefit of both modalities (Knobloch K., Kraemer R., 2015). Their biological "entry points," however, are not identical. Radial shockwaves, because

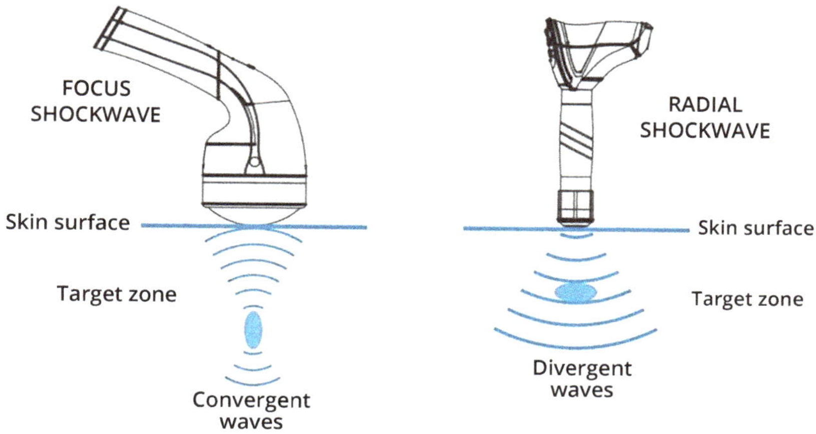

Fig. IV-3-6. Shockwave propagation in different types of shockwave therapy (https://www.kaphaphysio.com)

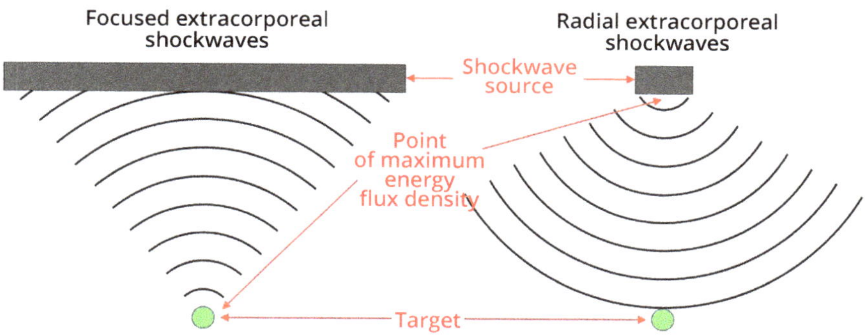

Fig. IV-3-7. Energy distribution in different shockwave therapy modalities

they deliver energy to soft tissues efficiently and are less affected by intervening structures, are often discussed for improving perfusion, supporting metabolism, and promoting lipolysis. Focused shockwaves, in contrast, act most strongly at the focal point and may directly injure adipocytes there, leading to apoptosis.

3.2.3. Shockwave therapy in complex anti-cellulite programs

Shockwave therapy can be used on its own, but it also pairs well with many other body-contouring methods. In combined protocols, it is often selected to reinforce lipolytic and lifting effects and to support lymphatic drainage. A few examples:

Duncan D.I. (2021) described a combined protocol combining HIFEM, RF, and focused shockwave therapy to address cellulite and improve the appearance of the abdomen and buttocks. The study included 15 participants (mean age 44.3 years; mean BMI ~22.3), divided into two treatment areas: Group 1 (abdomen; *N* = 7) and Group 2 (buttocks; *N* = 7). Participants received four 50-minute sessions, delivered twice weekly. The therapy had two stages: HIFEM first, followed by combined RF and focused shockwave therapy offered at the same visit. Clinical assessments were performed at three time points: baseline (before the course), 1 month after the course, and 3 months after completion. At the 1-month follow-up, participants showed a 4.4 cm decrease in abdominal circumference and a 1.0 cm increase in buttock circumference; these changes remained essentially unchanged at 3 months. Most participants (93.3%) reported being very satisfied, noting visible improvement in appearance, firmness, and overall skin quality. In summary, the multimodal protocol was described as safe, comfortable, and effective for contour refinement and skin improvement in the treated areas.

Allam N.M. et al. (2021) compared manual lymphatic drainage massage with radial shockwave therapy in post-liposuction patients with concerns about cellulite. The study enrolled 30 women with grade 3 cellulite and assigned them to two equal groups: Group 1 received shockwave therapy only, and Group 2 received massage only. Cellulite severity and SAT thickness were evaluated before treatment and again after 4 weeks. Improvement was significantly greater in the shockwave group.

Evidence also suggests that pairing shockwave therapy with aerobic exercise can further reduce cellulite severity on the buttocks and upper thighs in young women. Troia S. et al. (2021) studied 45 healthy women ages 18–32 and divided them into three groups: aerobic exercise alone, aerobic exercise plus radial shockwave therapy, and a no-intervention control. The combined-treatment group showed a significantly greater reduction in cellulite severity than either the exercise-only or the control group.

3.3. Gel for ultrasound and shockwave treatments

Conductive gel is a core part of ultrasound and shockwave treatments because it supports efficient energy transfer and helps keep sessions comfortable and safe. When used correctly, it improves both treatment performance and patient experience.

The gel's main job is to ensure reliable acoustic coupling between the handpiece and the skin. In practical terms, it reduces energy loss at the surface, enabling ultrasound or shockwaves to be delivered into tissue more predictably and effectively.

Additional roles include:

- Reducing resistance and friction, improving comfort during the procedure
- Promoting more uniform energy distribution across the treated area
- Protecting the skin from mechanical irritation when the handpiece is in contact with the surface;
- Improving contact consistency and helping maintain stable delivery during the session

Most gels are water-based and use polymers such as glycerol, carbomer, and polyvinyl alcohol. Water provides acoustic conductivity, while the polymers create the viscosity needed for even spread and good adherence to skin. Preservatives are essential for limiting microbial growth and maintaining product safety throughout the shelf life. Some formulations also include essential oils or antiseptics to enhance protection or support preventive use.

Technique matters. In most cases, a 3–5 mm layer is sufficient, which corresponds to about 20–40 g per treatment zone. The exact amount depends on the area size and the manufacturer's instructions.

Apply the gel evenly (with a spatula or directly from the tube), then spread it gently to thoroughly cover the surface. Place the handpiece against the skin with light, steady pressure so the gel distributes evenly, air gaps are eliminated, and wave transmission remains consistent. If the gel dries out or is removed during the session, reapply as needed to maintain proper coupling.

Chapter 4
Light technologies

4.1. Interaction of light with biological tissues

In light-assisted technologies, the active factor is light — electromagnetic radiation detectable by the human eye. Familiar light sources include lasers, intense pulsed light (IPL), and LEDs. They differ in both design and emission spectrum. Lasers deliver the narrowest output (essentially a single wavelength), LEDs emit a slightly broader yet still relatively limited band, and IPL covers the widest spectral range. Each approach has strengths and trade-offs, so choosing the best option depends on the clinical goal.

Light affects biological tissue through several core mechanisms:

1. **Photothermal effects:** When light is absorbed by tissue (more specifically, by the chromophores it contains), its energy is converted into heat. Depending on dose and target, this can produce substantial heating, protein coagulation, water vaporization, and even ablation (removal of tissue layers). Many surgical and aesthetic laser applications rely on this principle.
2. **Photomechanical (photoacoustic) effects:** High-intensity, short-pulse light can generate mechanical waves within tissue. These waves can disrupt cellular and extracellular structures with minimal overall heating. A classic example is laser lithotripsy, which fragments kidney stones.
3. **Photochemical reactions:** When chromophores absorb light, chemical reactions may be initiated. This mechanism underlies, for example, photostimulation of vitamin D production in the skin and photodynamic therapy, where light activates drugs that selectively damage target cells.

4. **Photobiological effects:** Light can modulate cellular and tissue biology, influencing proliferation, migration, inflammation, and immune responses. Low-intensity laser therapy, for instance, is used to support wound healing and reduce pain.
5. **Optical properties of tissues:** Different tissues vary in absorption, scattering, and reflection. These properties determine how deeply light penetrates and which structures receive the most significant exposure.

The biological effect — and therefore the clinical outcome — is shaped by several practical variables, including:

- Wavelengtht
- Radiation intensity
- Exposure duration
- The optical properties of the tissue
- The presence and concentration of chromophores in the target zone

Understanding these interactions enables the design and application of light-based methods for both diagnostic and therapeutic purposes, including aesthetic applications such as fat reduction and body contouring.

4.2. Laser lipolysis as an alternative to traditional liposuction

In 1999, Dr. Rodrigo Neira and colleagues published a paper suggesting that low-intensity laser exposure can emulsify adipose tissue (Neira R. et al., 2002). In their work, light at 635 nm was shown to create temporary pores in adipocyte membranes, allowing lipid content to exit the cell. This finding helped spark the development of laser lipolysis — a body-contouring approach that differs from traditional liposuction, where fat is mechanically disrupted and then aspirated.

After this publication, interest grew in using light energy to selectively affect adipose tissue. Early reports suggested that laser-based approaches could support fat removal while sparing surrounding structures, potentially leading to less discomfort and faster recovery (Bellini E. et al., 2017). Key milestones in the field include:

- **2006:** A significant step forward came with the FDA clearance of the first laser system designed specifically for laser lipolysis. SmartLipo (Cynosure), based on a 1064 nm Nd:YAG laser, marked the formal entry of laser technology into clinical liposuction and supported wider adoption in US aesthetic practice.
- **2007:** The 1320 nm laser was introduced and showed improved fat liquefaction alongside collagen stimulation, highlighting that laser lipolysis could contribute not only to fat reduction but also to overall skin quality.
- **2009:** Hybrid systems emitting two wavelengths (1064 nm and 1320 nm) became available. Dual-wavelength delivery enabled more flexible treatment planning, targeting both more profound and more superficial fat while supporting dermal collagen remodeling.
- **2012:** Diode lasers at 1470 nm entered the market for laser lipolysis. Because this wavelength is absorbed more efficiently by water and fat, it improved both efficacy and the safety profile.
- **2015:** The FDA cleared 1060 nm diode lasers for non-invasive fat reduction, further expanding the role of laser-based options in body contouring.

4.3. Laser lipolysis technologies: variants and effects

Laser lipolysis is built around selective photothermolysis, where light at a specific wavelength is used to target adipose tissue preferentially.

4.3.1. "Hot" laser lipolysis

In "hot" laser lipolysis, the primary working mechanism is controlled heating of the target zone. Within the 400–1500 nm range, adipose tissue shows several absorption peaks — notably at 924 nm, 1064 nm,

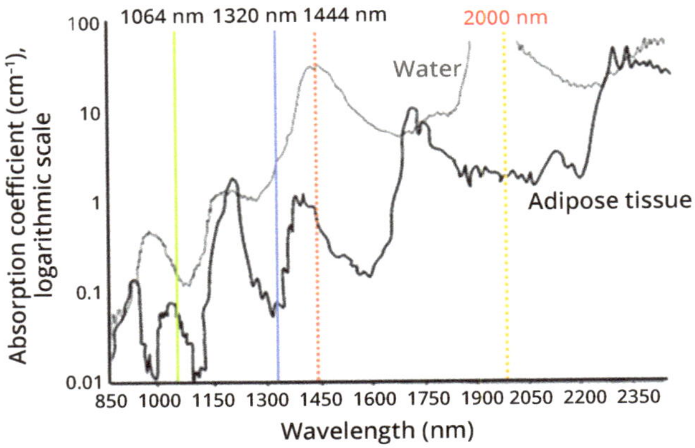

Fig. IV-4-1. Absorption coefficients of human adipose tissue and water (adapted from Lee J.Y. et al., 2021; CC BY)

1210 nm, and 1440 nm (**Fig. IV-4-1**). In practical terms, wavelengths closer to these peaks are absorbed more readily, enabling rapid heating of fat cells. This can lead to thermal injury and release of lipid material into the extracellular space.

At the same time, water also absorbs strongly in this optical range, which contributes to volumetric heating of tissue. As temperature rises, collagen fibers change their spatial arrangement, affecting both the fibrous septa within SAT and the collagen-elastin framework in the dermis. Clinically, this may produce post-procedure skin flap contraction at the treatment site, although the effect is temporary. More importantly, portions of collagen become irreversibly denatured and more vulnerable to proteolytic enzymes. This triggers breakdown of damaged collagen, followed by replacement with newly synthesized collagen, resulting in tissue remodeling (Lee J.Y. et al., 2021).

When selecting a wavelength, depth of penetration is a key consideration. In general, longer wavelengths tend to reach deeper — but this relationship weakens as wavelengths approach 2000 nm, where water absorption becomes pronounced (**Fig. IV-4-2**).

To reduce burn risk, it is essential to keep the skin surface temperature below 40–47 °C — the range associated with adipocyte death — while temperatures of 48–54 °C are typically required to produce irreversible adipocyte injury and collagen denaturation within SAT.

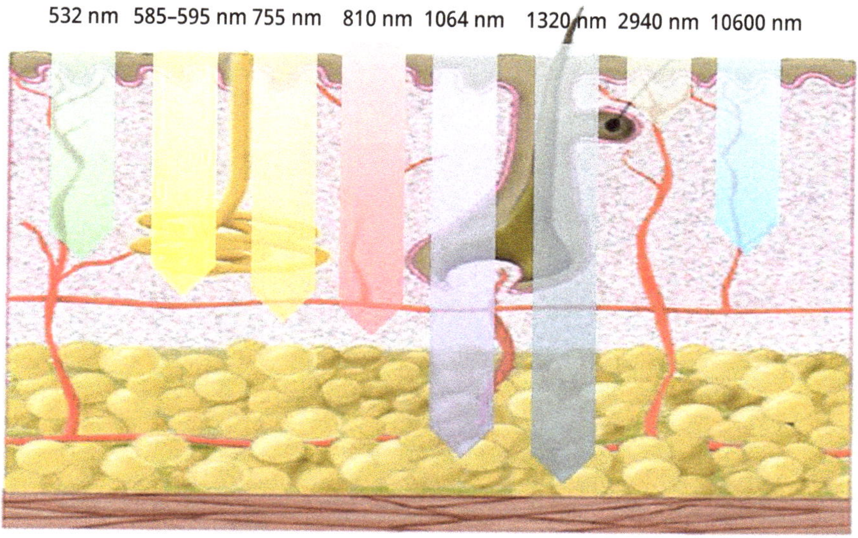

Fig. IV-4-2. Depth of light penetration in the skin (adapted from Lee J.Y. et al., 2021; CC BY)

Minimally invasive laser lipolysis and laser-assisted liposuction

In the minimally invasive approach to laser lipolysis, light energy is delivered directly into the target zone. The most commonly used options are Nd:YAG lasers at 1064 nm, although 1320 nm and 1440 nm systems are also available (Manzano-Finol A. et al., 2025). Multi-wavelength platforms that combine two or even three wavelengths are another option. For example, SmartLipo® Triplex® (Cynosure Lutronic, USA) is an Nd:YAG laser that operates at 1064 nm, 1320 nm, and 1440 nm. Energy can be delivered in single-wavelength or blended modes. According to the manufacturer's description, flexible parameter selection supports efficient fat liquefaction and visible skin retraction, while helping lower the likelihood of adverse events such as burns, bleeding, or hematomas.

Through a small incision, a cannula of about 1 mm in diameter is introduced with an optical fiber inside it (**Fig. IV-4-3**). The fiber is advanced through the cannula, so its working tip extends about 2–3 mm beyond the cannula. When the laser is activated, heating

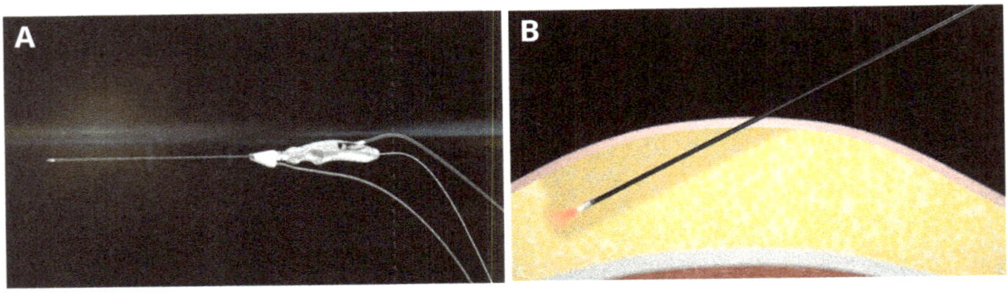

Fig. IV-4-3. Optical fiber cannula for minimally invasive lipolysis: A — cannula; B — heating focus at the cannula tip (Photo: SmartLipo®Triplex®/ Cynosure Lutronic, USA; https://www.cynosure.com/product/smartlipo-triplex)

is concentrated near this exposed tip; clinically, the treatment point can be tracked because the light transilluminates through the skin. The emulsified fat is then aspirated through the probe, which is why this technique is commonly referred to as **laser-assisted liposuction** (Ali Y.H., 2018).

Temperature is monitored at multiple tissue depths using dedicated sensors, and if overheating is detected, energy delivery is stopped (Kosir J. et al., 2020). Light may be delivered continuously or in pulses. Pulsed delivery is often preferred because it can disrupt adipocytes efficiently while keeping burn risk low. Parameters are selected based on the treatment area. For example, Piccolo D. et al. (2023) reported the following settings for a 1444 nm Nd:YAG (LipoAI/ Deka M.e.l.a, Italy):

- Face: Power 5–6 W, Frequency 20–30 Hz, Energy 800–1500 J
- Body: Power 6–7 W, Frequency 30–40 Hz, Energy 1000–3500 J

Non-invasive laser lipolysis

Laser lipolysis can also be performed non-invasively — using a 1060 nm GaAs diode laser (Decorato J. et al., 2017; Schilling L. et al., 2017; Kwon T.R. et al., 2021). During treatment, the skin is actively cooled to maintain a surface temperature of 15 °C. Adipocytes affected within the hyperemic zone are cleared through normal metabolic pathways, and the local inflammatory response recruits macrophages to remove cellular debris.

4.3.2 "Cold" laser lipolysis

Non-invasive laser lipolysis, often marketed as "cold lipolysis" or a "cold laser", uses low-intensity laser irradiation (LLLI) in the red or near-infrared range. Most diode systems operate between 635 nm and 980 nm, although longer wavelengths may also be used. Because power levels are far lower than in traditional laser procedures (mW/cm^2 vs. W/cm^2), there is essentially no meaningful heating in the treated area.

The exact mechanism by which LLLI affects adipose tissue remains unclear. Early studies proposed that temporary micropores form in adipocyte membranes, allowing lipids to exit the cell and enter the extracellular space. Later concepts suggested that LLLI may activate the complement cascade and, in turn, trigger apoptosis in adipocytes. Another hypothesis focuses on mitochondrial respiration: if LLLI increases mitochondrial activity, it may raise ATP levels and also increase cAMP, which can enhance cytoplasmic lipase activity and promote triglyceride breakdown into free fatty acids and glycerol. At the same time, greater mitochondrial activity can generate more reactive oxygen species (ROS), which are natural byproducts of oxygen-dependent ATP production. These ROS may contribute to membrane lipid peroxidation and ultimately adipocyte death (Nishioka M.A. et al., 2025).

It is important to emphasize that none of these mechanisms has been definitively proven. Still, published studies report reductions in fat-depot volume (Jackson R.F. et al., 2012; Savoia A. et al., 2013) and histologic changes in irradiated tissue, including inflammatory-cell infiltration (for example, CD68+ macrophages), consistent with clearance of adipocyte fragments from the treated area (Modena D.A.O. et al., 2022; Nishioka M.A. et al., 2025).

Across studies, authors repeatedly note that outcomes are more reliable when non-invasive laser lipolysis is paired with measures that support microcirculation and lymphatic drainage, along with regular physical activity and appropriate nutrition. Irradiation can be delivered using handpieces placed directly on the skin (for example, iLipo/Chromogenex, UK; **Fig. IV-4-4**) or via non-contact delivery (for example, Zerona/Erchonia, USA; **Fig. IV-4-5**).

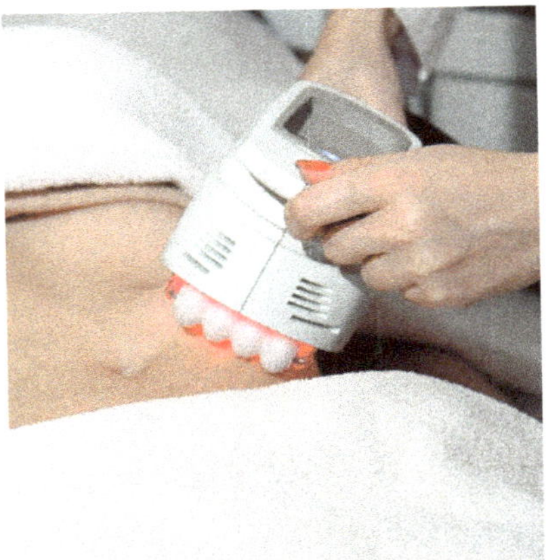

Fig. IV-4-4. Contact "cold" laser lipolysis

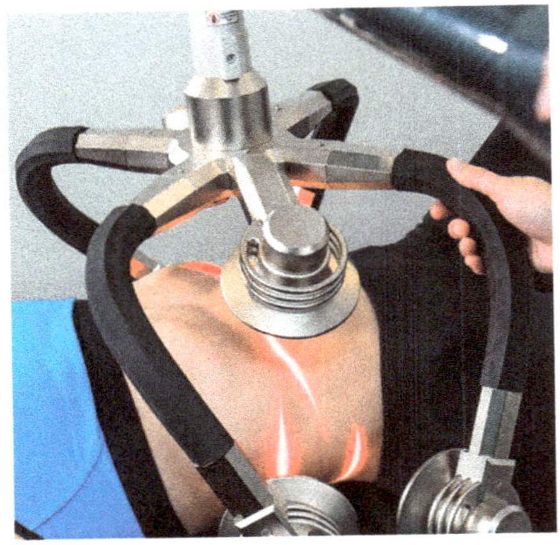

Fig. IV-4-5. Non-contact "cold" lase lipolysis

On average, a session lasts about 40–60 min. Afterward, a lymphatic drainage massage is commonly recommended (about 30 min to 1.5 hours). The procedure is painless, and no adverse effects have been reported. The total number of sessions is individualized, but most protocols include 6–12 procedures spaced 1–2 days apart. Results are often noted within a week after completing the course.

Best candidates tend to be healthy individuals with small, localized fat deposits, as well as patients with obesity and hormonal factors who may have contraindications to other lipolytic approaches.

Chapter 5
Cryolipolysis

Cryolipolysis is a non-invasive approach to reducing SAT volume that leverages adipocytes' selective sensitivity to cold. With prolonged, localized cooling — typically for about 1 hour — fat cells can be injured and ultimately eliminated without harming other skin cells. Adipocyte loss occurs through apoptosis and develops gradually over several weeks after the procedure. Importantly, this process does not produce an acute inflammatory reaction or a significant, sudden release of breakdown products into the blood and lymphatic systems.

Cryolipolysis entered aesthetic medicine in 2009 and quickly became popular because it combined noticeable results with a favorable safety profile and minimal downtime. Soon after, however, reports of unexpected adverse effects — most notably paradoxical hyperplasia of adipose tissue (PHA) — tempered early enthusiasm.

Today, cryolipolysis remains widely used to treat cellulite and localized fat deposits, with newer systems and refined protocols aimed at reducing risk. The U.S. Food and Drug Administration (FDA) has approved cryolipolysis for treating visible fat deposits in the subchin (submental) and submandibular areas, the back, upper arms, thighs, abdomen, flanks, and the area beneath the buttocks.

5.1. Historical background

The idea of using low temperatures to address excessive fat deposits emerged from clinical observation (Jalian H.R., Avram M.M., 2013). In the early 20th century, physicians described cases of cold panniculitis (adiponecrosis subcutanea) — an acute inflammatory response of SAT to cold. Clinically, it presents as firm, red nodules that typically appear 1–2 days after cold exposure. Lesions most often occur in exposed areas with relatively prominent SAT, such as the cheeks and chin. During generalized hypothermia, similar changes can also appear elsewhere (Greenwald E. et al., 2018).

The first report is commonly attributed to Austrian pediatrician Carl Hochsinger in 1902. He described firm submental nodules in children aged 4–10 and linked them to an acute response to cold (Hochsinger C., 1902). In 1941, Holger Haxthausen, a pediatric dermatologist in Copenhagen, published a case series he termed "adiponecrosis e frigore" — "adiponecrosis of freezing" (Haxthausen H., 1941). His report included four young children and one adolescent who developed skin findings similar to those of Hochsinger after exposure to severe winter cold. Between 1940 and 1970, multiple publications described red, firm nodules consistent with cold panniculitis following prolonged exposure to intense cold in both children and adults. In 1970, American physicians Ervin H. Epstein and Mark E. Oren introduced the term "popsicle panniculitis" after observing similar cheek changes in a child following ice cream exposure.

These clinical patterns suggested that lipid-rich tissues respond differently to cold than water-rich tissues. Because infants and young children were affected more often than adults, researchers proposed that adipose sensitivity might depend on the balance of saturated and unsaturated fatty acids (Adams J.E. et al., 1955). In adults, subcutaneous fat contains up to 40% saturated fatty acids and up to 60% unsaturated fatty acids. In infants and young children, SAT contains a higher proportion of saturated fatty acids, including palmitic and stearic acids (Quesada-Cortés A. et al., 2008). Saturated fats have higher melting points than unsaturated fats, which influences whether the lipid phase is more solid or liquid at a given temperature. The greater the saturated fraction, the more readily fat "freezes" and becomes denser — a change that can compromise cell viability.

In 2008, a research team at Harvard Medical School (Boston, USA), led by Dr. Dieter Manstein — who later proposed the term "cryolipolysis" — published a series of porcine experiments (Manstein D. et al., 2008). To test localized cold exposure on SAT, a skin fold was cooled to –1 to –8 °C for 10 min, followed by histologic evaluation at 3.5 months. The authors found that cooling induced focal panniculitis and, over time, a marked reduction in the fat layer at the treated site.

In 2009, these experiments were extended using the CoolSculpting cryolipolysis system developed by Zeltiq® Aesthetics (acquired by Allergan, USA, in 2017). The study was performed in pigs at –7 °C with exposure times of 45–60 min. Manstein and colleagues showed that cold exposure could significantly reduce the superficial fat layer without injuring the epidermis or dermis. Averaged across animals, fat-layer thickness decreased by approximately 30% (Zelickson B. et al., 2009).

5.2. Cryolipolysis technologies: variants and effects

SAT cooling can be achieved in two main ways: with cryolipolysis systems or by injecting ice chips. In this chapter, we focus on system-based cryolipolysis; ice injections are covered in the section on injectable lipodestruction (see Part V, section 1.2.2).

5.2.1. Vacuum-assisted cryolipolysis

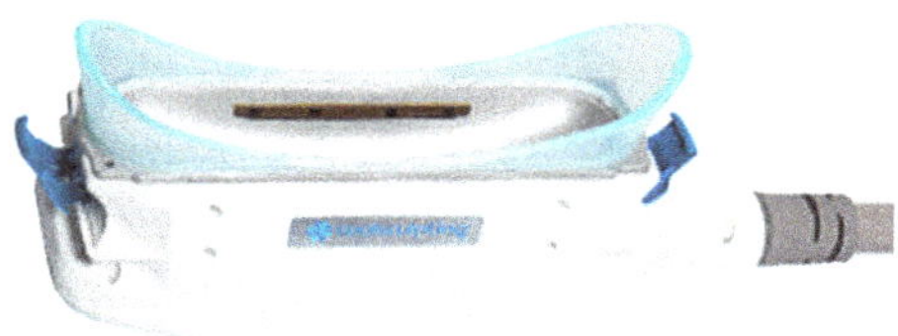

Fig. IV-5-1. A dome-shaped cryolipolysis handpiece (CoolSculpting handpiece shown as an example)

Vacuum-assisted cryolipolysis is the standard method. Localized cooling of SAT is delivered using a dome-shaped handpiece. A soft gasket along the rim creates an airtight seal between the handpiece and the skin (**Fig. IV-5-1**). Handpieces come in different sizes to match different body areas and contours. Most modern cryolipolysis systems include a set of handpieces in multiple sizes (**Fig. IV 5-2**). Many also offer interchangeable gaskets of different heights, allowing even closer matching to the topography of the target zone (**Fig. IV-5-3**).

During treatment, negative pressure inside the handpiece draws a skin fold into the cup, where it is cooled by heat-exchanging elements (**Fig. IV-5-4**).

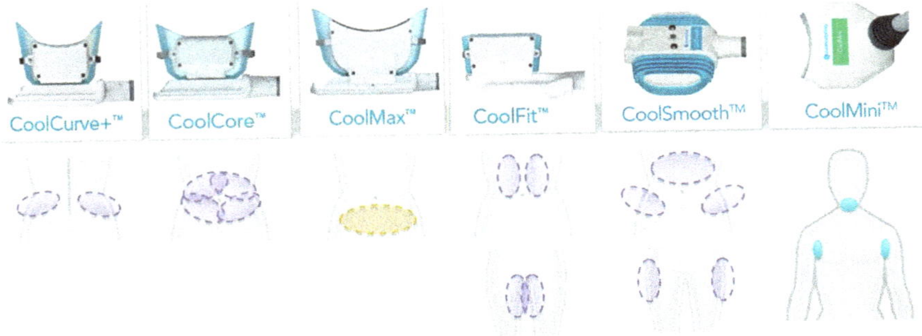

Fig. IV-5-2. Cryolipolysis handpieces are adapted to different body areas (CoolSculpting system shown as an example)

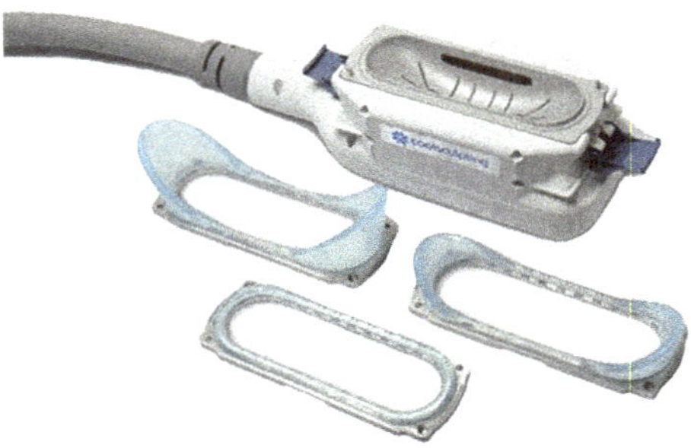

Fig. IV-5-3. Interchangeable contours for a dome-shaped cryolipolysis handpiece (CoolSculpting handpiece shown as an example)

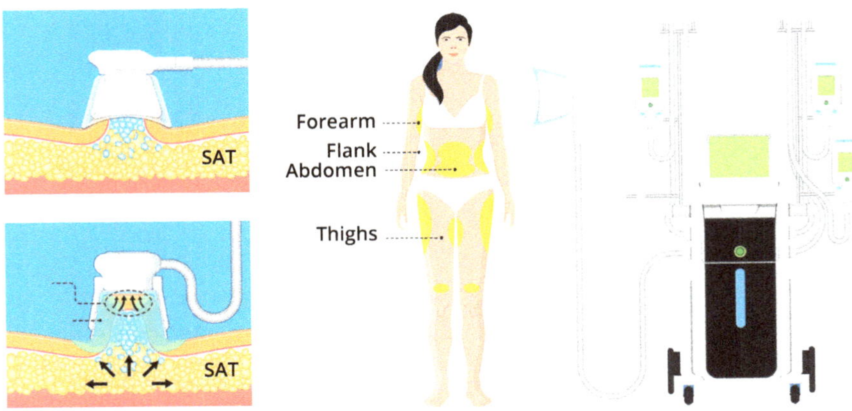

Fig. IV-5-4. Principle of vacuum-assisted cryolipolysis (Image: Papermpron / Shutterstock)

Three main mechanisms are typically used to explain the reduction in localized fat:

1. **Fat crystallization and direct mechanical injury to adipocytes.** Vacuum suction combined with controlled cooling reduces local blood flow and promotes lipid crystallization at the exposure site, which can directly injure adipocytes. Because lipids transition into a solid phase at higher temperatures than water (about +10 °C vs. 0 °C), cooling can selectively affect fat cells while leaving water-dominant cells relatively intact. Solid lipid crystals may mechanically disrupt adipocytes and cause necrosis, or initiate apoptosis by impairing membrane-associated enzymes (Manstein D. et al., 2008).
2. **Activation of apoptotic pathways in adipocytes.** Cold ischemic injury can amplify adipocyte damage by disrupting key biochemical processes, including those involved in membrane enzyme dysfunction. For example, reduced Na^+/K^+-ATPase activity contributes to cellular swelling. Impaired enzyme activity on the inner mitochondrial membrane — where ATP production is regulated — can disrupt energy-dependent processes and promote intracellular acidosis as lactic acid accumulates (Belzer F.O., Southard J.H., 1988). Because SAT white adipocytes contain relatively few mitochondria, even modest mitochondrial dysfunction can have outsized effects.
3. **Oxidative stress is associated with reperfusion.** Injury initiated by crystallization and ischemia during the procedure may be compounded afterward by ischemia-reperfusion injury. Reperfusion — the restoration of blood flow to previously ischemic tissue — causes a sudden rise in oxygen availability. This drives mitochondrial respiration upward and can sharply increase ROS production, triggering rapid intracellular oxidative stress (Sakon M. et al., 2002). ROS is a natural by-product of mitochondrial oxidative metabolism; the more intense the respiration, the more ROS is generated. Under normal conditions, antioxidant defenses keep ROS in check. After cold ischemia, however, these defenses may be insufficient to buffer a sudden ROS surge, and oxidative stress can help push cells toward apoptosis.

By the day after the procedure, increased numbers of adipocytes with morphologic signs of apoptosis are typically observed in the cold-ischemia zone. At the same time, inflammatory cells — neutrophils, lymphocytes, and monocytes — accumulate locally, producing a mild inflammatory response. This response peaks toward the end of the first week (D7) and subsides by the end of the second week (D15). By the end of the first month, active phagocytosis of adipocyte debris becomes evident, and patients may begin to notice early visible changes (Meyer P.F. et al., 2016).

Beyond adipocyte loss, the fibrous septa also undergo structural change. Ultrasound suggests connective-tissue remodeling occurs in stages: at peak inflammation (D7), septa appear thinner; as inflammation resolves (D15), septa thicken, and features of fibrosis emerge. By D30, fibrosis is minimal, and septa look thinner again. At about 1.5 months (D45), fibrotic changes can reappear, though typically less pronounced, and septa measure thicker than baseline (**Table IV-5-1**). Macroscopic assessment confirms fat-layer thinning (**Fig. IV-5-5**), while histology demonstrates corresponding structural changes (**Fig. IV-5-6**) (Meyer P.F. et al., 2016).

Table IV-5-1. SAT and fibrous septum thickness based on ultrasound findings (Meyer P.F. et al., 2016)

	AVERAGE THICKNESS (cm)				
	BEFORE	D7	D15	D30	D45
SAT	3.67	2.59	2.57	2.41	2.21
Fibrous septa	0.10	0.06	0.66	0.16	0.22

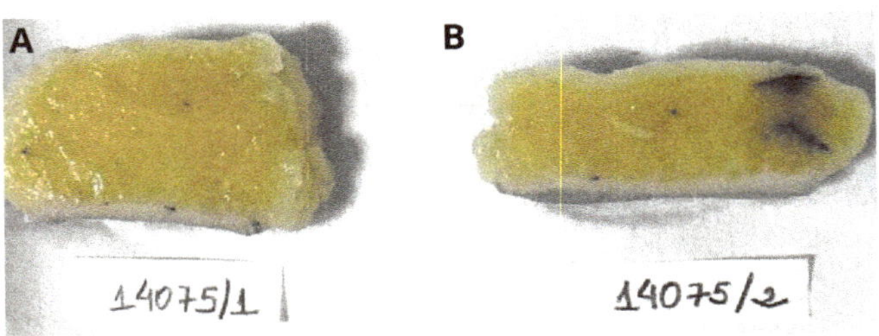

Fig. IV-5-5: Macroscopic assessment of tissue collected during abdominoplasty: A — untreated side (546 g; 15 × 10 cm); B — treated side (508 g; 15 × 10 cm) (adapted from Meyer P.F. et al., 2016; CC BY)

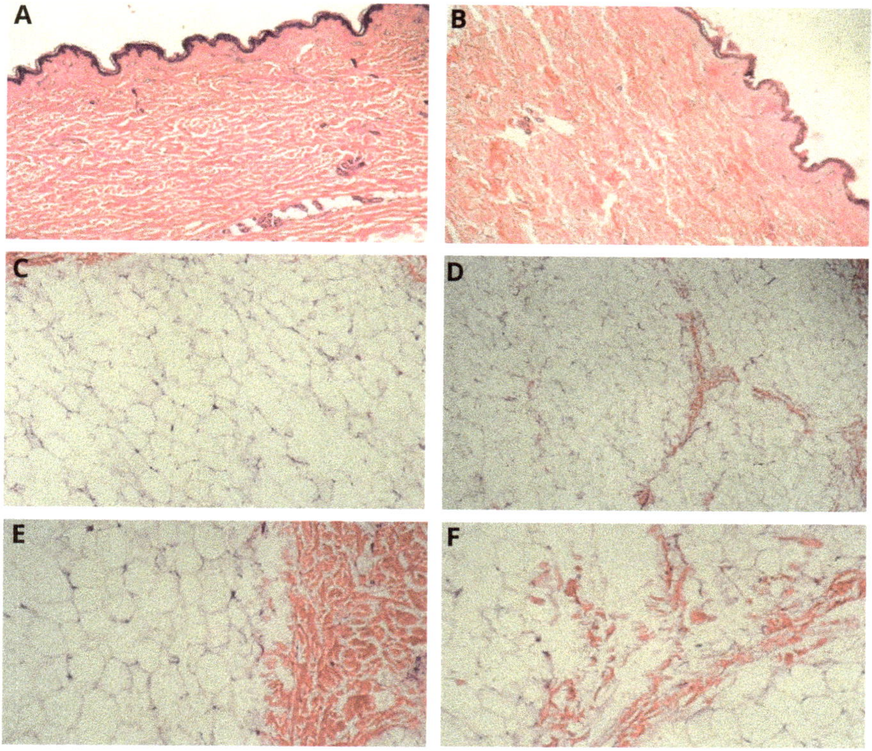

Fig. IV-5-6. Microscopic analysis of tissue collected during abdominoplasty. Longitudinal sections, hematoxylin-eosin staining: (100x) untreated area (A) and treated area (B); (100x) adipocyte membrane disruption and fibrosis in the mid-layer of adipose tissue (B, D); (400x) treated area with preserved adjacent tissue and fibrosis in the mid-layer of adipose tissue (E, F) (adapted from Meyer P.F. et al., 2016; CC BY)

On average, fat-layer thickness decreases by about 20% after a single session (Meyer P.F. et al., 2016; Silva G.A.T. et al., 2021). Outcomes are typically assessed at 90 days.

More recent work has also reported "browning" of white adipose tissue in response to abrupt cold exposure (see Part I, section 1.2). This may be an additional contributor to reduced SAT volume (Gao Y. et al., 2018; Qiu J. et al., 2023).

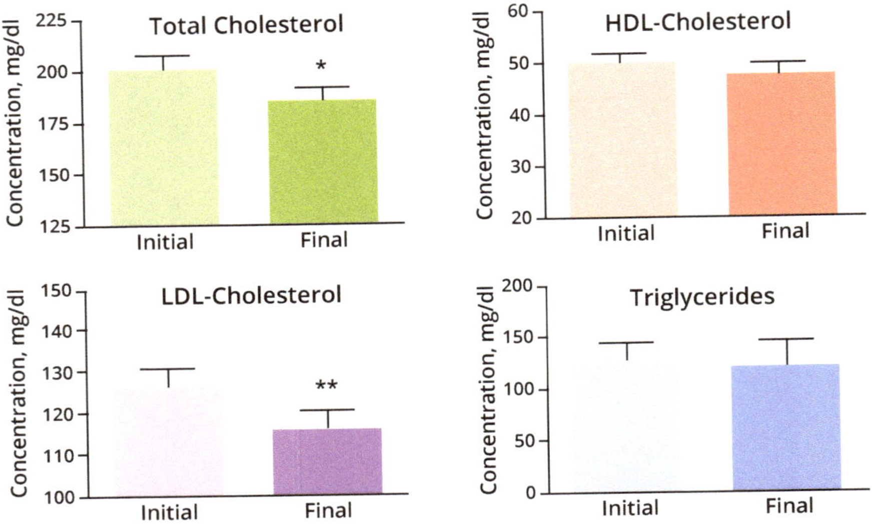

Fig. IV-5-7. Mean and standard deviation of plasma lipids before and after three cryolipolysis sessions. Patients: women with high BMI and obesity (n = 30). A p-value was considered significant if it was ≤ 0.05. (* $p \leq 0.05$; ** $p \leq 0.01$) (adapted from Lopes-Martins R.A.B. et al., 2024; CC BY)

Because apoptosis unfolds gradually, cryolipolysis does not produce dramatic short-term or long-term shifts in blood lipids, glucose, or liver enzymes (Ingargiola M.J. et al., 2015; Klein K.B. et al., 2017). Some recent studies have even reported reductions in cholesterol after multiple cryolipolysis sessions, suggesting potential value in broader health-focused programs for patients with obesity, diabetes, or cardiovascular disease (**Fig. IV-5-7**) (Lopes-Martins R.A.B. et al., 2024).

In this context, findings from Hwang I.C. et al. (2020) are exciting because they examined effects on both subcutaneous and visceral abdominal fat. The study enrolled 15 participants (9 women and 6 men) with a mean age of 38.3 years. Each participant underwent a single cryolipolysis session on the left abdomen, with the right side serving as a control. Cross-sectional areas of abdominal adipose tissue were measured by computed tomography at baseline and 12 weeks post-treatment (**Fig. IV-5-8**). Waist circumference and

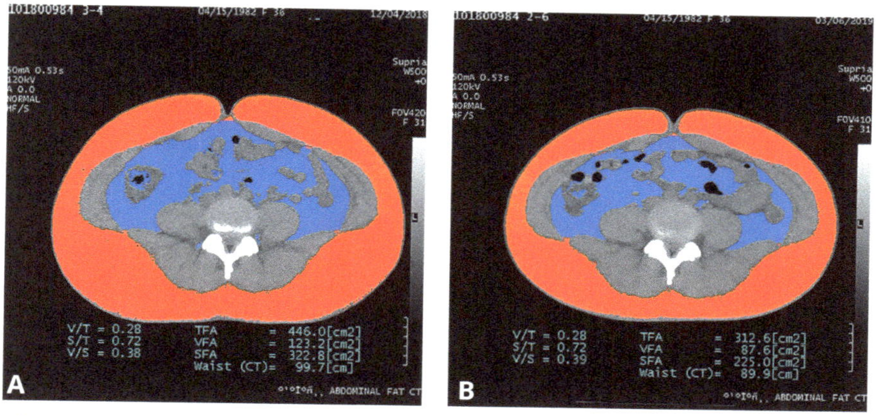

Fig. IV-5-8. Cross-sectional area of visceral and subcutaneous adipose tissue: A — baseline; B — after 12 weeks (subcutaneous fat in red, visceral fat in blue). Left — untreated side (control); right — treated side (adapted from Hwang I.C. et al., 2020; CC BY)

body-fat percentage (via bioimpedance) were recorded at baseline and again at 6 and 12 weeks.

After one session, the authors reported a trend toward reductions in visceral fat cross-sectional area (by 8.4 cm^2, or 9.9%), waist circumference (by 2.8 cm), and body-fat percentage (by 0.6%). Notably, visceral fat on the treated side decreased significantly (by 6.8 cm^2, or 15.6%), while the untreated side also showed a more minor reduction (by 1.2 cm^2, or 3.6%). These results suggest cryolipolysis may have a role beyond purely aesthetic goals, potentially fitting into weight-management programs by affecting both subcutaneous and visceral compartments. The observation of change on the control side also raises the question of broader metabolic effects after localized cooling — an area where additional research is clearly needed.

5.2.2. Contrast cryolipolysis

One variation of vacuum-assisted cryolipolysis is contrast cryolipolysis. In this protocol, the fat layer is heated before and after cold exposure (**Fig. IV-5-9**). RF current is commonly used for the heating

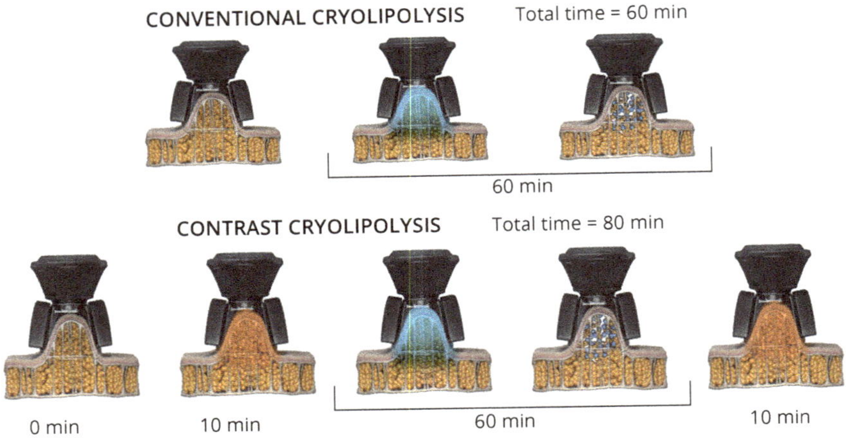

Fig. IV-5-9. Classic cryolipolysis vs. contrast cryolipolysis (adapted from Savacini M.B. et al., 2018; CC BY)

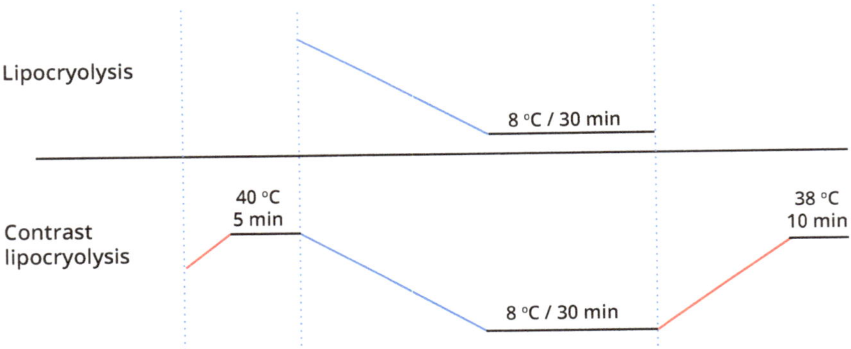

Fig. IV-5-10. Target tissue temperature in classic vs. contrast cryolipolysis (adapted from Pinto H., Melamed G., 2012; CC BY)

When the temperature is below 36 °C, blood flow naturally accelerates, producing an average heating rate of 8.25 °C/min (red line). At around 36 °C, blood flow limits further heating, and the average heating rate drops to 2 °C/min. The cooling rate (blue line) is 3 °C/min. Target temperature in adipocytes (black line): 40 °C for 5 min (pre-cooling), < 10 °C for 30 min (cryolipolysis), and 38 °C for 10 min (recovery). Total duration of the contrast protocol was 60 min.

phase (Savacini M.B. et al., 2018). This temperature contrast appears to intensify adipose-tissue injury, likely due in part to how blood flow influences tissue temperature and to temperature-dependent cellular processes (**Fig. IV-5-10**) (Pinto H., Melamed G., 2014).

5.2.3 Cryolipolysis with plates

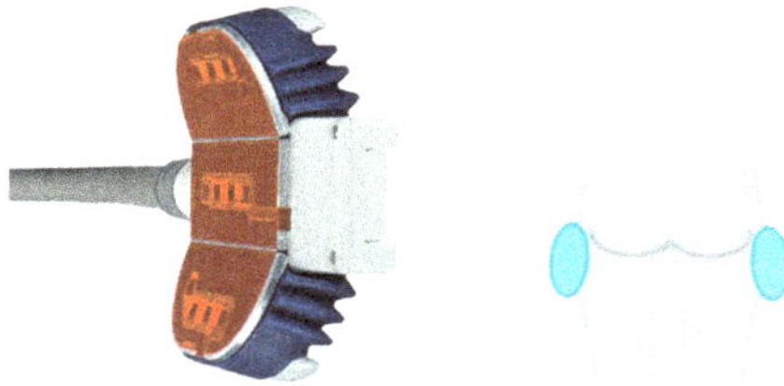

Fig. IV-5-11. Plate handpiece for the saddlebag area (CoolSculpting handpiece shown as an example)

Some cryolipolysis systems use plate applicators that cool the skin fold through surface contact. Treatment with these applicators is usually more comfortable than protocols that rely on vacuum suction (Stevens W.G., Bachelor E.P., 2015). The trade-off is that, without tissue ischemia and with ongoing blood flow, it can be harder to maintain uniform cooling in the deeper layers of the fold, potentially reducing overall efficacy.

That said, plate applicators can be a good practical choice for areas such as the "saddlebag" region, where forming a sufficiently thin fold can be challenging (**Fig. IV-5-11**).

5.2.4. Electromyostimulation + cooling

Some systems combine EMS with cooling (**Fig. IV-5-12**). Their handpiece includes electrodes for EMS and a surface-cooling module. Because the handpiece is placed on the skin without drawing a fold into a vacuum cup — and without creating ischemia — it cannot reliably deliver the low temperatures needed to destroy adipocytes deep within the fold. As a result, changes in SAT, if present, are usually minimal.

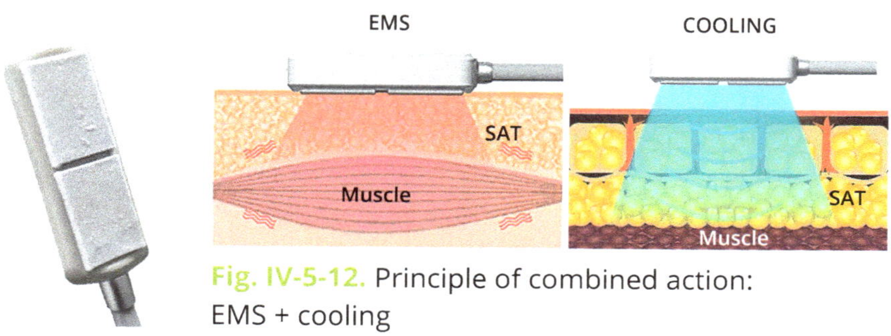

Fig. IV-5-12. Principle of combined action: EMS + cooling

At the same time, because EMS is involved, an effect on visceral fat may be expected (see Part IV, section 2.6.4). This is why such systems are often positioned as slimming solutions and are used primarily in the abdominal region.

5.3. Indications and contraindications

Indications

1. Excess fat deposits in the abdomen, flanks, back, and thighs (fold thickness of at least 2.5 cm and no more than 6 cm)
2. Fat deposits on the arms
3. Submental fullness ("second chin")
4. Obesity: hormonal, digestive system disease, psychological (stress eating)
5. Cellulite
6. Irregularities after liposuction or minimally invasive lipolysis
7. Lack of the desired effect from diet and sports

Contraindications

1. Violation of skin integrity (wounds, abrasions, ulcers)
2. Dermatologic diseases in the acute phase
3. Presence of extensive scars and hernias in the treatment area
4. Diseases of the hematopoietic system
5. Thrombosis
6. Increased fragility of blood vessels
7. Individual intolerance to cold
8. Obesity II and III degrees
9. Diabetes mellitus
10. Mental disorders
11. Renal and hepatic failure
12. Epilepsy
13. Pregnancy and breastfeeding
14. Infectious diseases
15. Presence of a pacemaker or defibrillator in the body
16. Thin SAT

5.4. Factors affecting efficacy

Cryolipolysis outcomes are typically judged by how much the fat layer thins — measured as the difference in thickness before treatment and at 2 months (**Table IV-5-2**). Results vary by treatment zone, which makes clinical sense: different fat depots differ in vascularization, cytoarchitecture, and metabolic activity.

Table IV-5-2. Cryolipolysis efficacy in different areas and patient satisfaction (Few J. et al., 2020)

ZONE	NUMBER OF SESSION	FOLLOW-UP PERIOD, MONTHS	CORRECT OBSERVATIONS (%)	CONCLUSION	PATIENT SATISFACTION (%)
Flanks	1–3	6	89	–19%	82
Abdomen	1–2	4	85	–1.9 mm	62
Inner surface of the thigh	1	4	91	–2.8 mm	93
Outer surface of the thigh	1	4	84	–2.5 mm	87
Submental zone	1–2	3	91	–2.0 mm (–20%)	83
Upper arm	1	3	85	–3.2 mm	63

In clinical practice, the most noticeable change is usually observed in patients with mild-to-moderate localized fat deposits and in those with cellulite (Few J. et al., 2020).

To set realistic expectations and maximize results, it helps to consider a combination of factors related to the patient and to the technology used.

5.4.1. Patient selection

An ideal candidate profile for cryolipolysis typically includes:

- No contraindications to surgery.
- Low BMI — ideally below 30 kg/m^2. Cryolipolysis is best suited for contour refinement and localized fat reduction, not for significant weight loss.
- Skin elasticity is normal to moderate. If skin is lax and inelastic, combining cryolipolysis with skin-remodeling procedures is often recommended to support tightening in the treated area.
- Request to treat zones that are prone to contour irregularities after liposuction. Cryolipolysis is often preferred for folds on the flanks, inner thighs, knees, and the back below the bra line because fascial septa in SAT can be relatively dense, and aspiration from lobules may be uneven during liposuction.
- Desire to avoid scarring. Cryolipolysis is non-invasive and does not leave scars.
- Desire to avoid downtime — recovery after cryolipolysis is typically fast.
- Inability or unwillingness to undergo surgery. Cryolipolysis may be an option for patients with contraindications to liposuction or those who cannot tolerate anesthesia.

5.4.2. Technical issues

Volume of cooled adipose tissue

The volume of cooled adipose tissue depends on:

1. **Size and number of handpieces.** A larger handpiece covers a larger surface area, which should improve efficacy. In practice, uniform cooling is harder to achieve in a large fold — temperature often ends up lower at the periphery than at the center. In addition, a large fold may maintain greater blood flow, bringing more heat into the tissue. For large zones such as the abdomen and flanks, using several smaller handpieces is often more effective than relying on one large handpiece (Bachelor E. et al., 2025).

2. **Strength of the suction.** Higher vacuum typically draws in more fat and increases ischemia, but it also tends to increase soreness.

Temperature in the exposure zone

Adipocyte apoptosis can be triggered at temperatures below +10 °C, and cooling to about +7 °C within the fat fold is often considered optimal. At the same time, the skin surface that contacts the cooling plates can reach much lower values, including subzero temperatures (**Fig. IV-5-13**). Skin can adapt well to cold, but avoiding necrosis requires strict adherence to temperature protocols: cooling plates should not drop below –10 °C, and the *stratum corneum* should be pretreated with propylene glycol to reduce the risk of ice-crust formation. A protective pad soaked in the same substance is placed between the handpiece and the skin to support even heat transfer.

Cryolipolysis systems are commonly described as either fixed-temperature or adjustable-temperature:

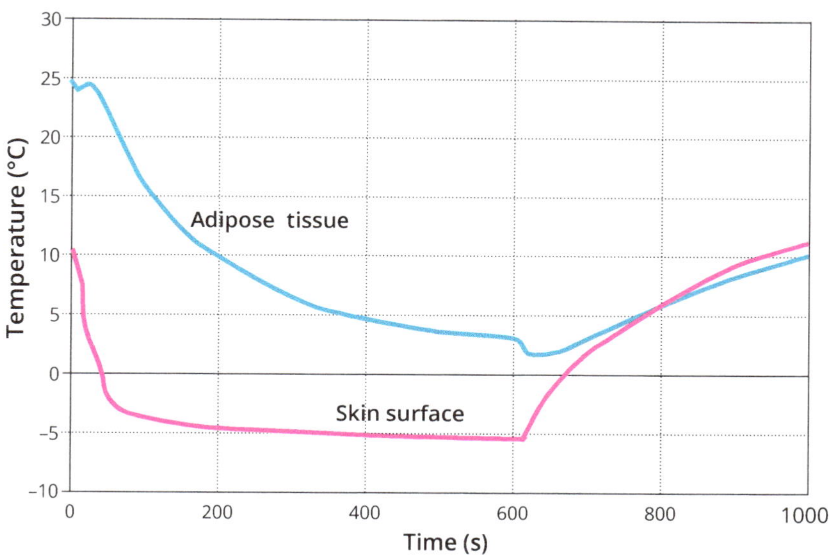

Fig. IV-5-13. Temperature at the skin surface and within the adipose layer during cooling of a skin fold (panel temperature –7 °C; session duration — 10 min) (adapted from Manstein D. et al., 2008; CC BY)

- **Fixed-temperature systems** follow a consistent protocol that supports a high safety margin, but they do not allow the operator to fine-tune intensity for efficacy.
- **Adjustable-temperature systems** use sensors and feedback control to maintain a target temperature and to stop cooling immediately if critical low thresholds are reached. This matters because internal tissue warming depends on the patient's anatomy and physiology.

Session duration

A cryolipolysis session typically lasts 30–60 min. Shorter exposure is generally considered insufficient to reach the temperature range associated with adipocyte apoptosis, while extending exposure beyond 1 hour does not reliably improve outcomes. Longer sessions also add discomfort, and patient tolerance becomes a practical limiting factor.

Number of treatments

IMultiple sessions in the same anatomical area can produce a more pronounced effect. However, each additional session often yields less incremental change than the previous one (Pinto H.R. et al., 2012; Shek S.Y. et al., 2012). Possible reasons include increased cold tolerance in surviving adipocytes and more effective internal warming of a thinning fat layer by underlying muscle (which is not captured within the suctioned fold), preventing the tissue from reaching apoptosis-triggering temperatures.

Mechanical effects

Mechanical manipulation can enhance outcomes. A 2-min manual massage immediately after cryolipolysis (1 min of vigorous kneading between the fingers and 1 min of circular massage) has been shown to significantly improve aesthetic results at 2 and 4 months (Boey G.E., Wasilenchuk J.L., 2014). Similar observations have been reported for mechanical massage performed for 5 min during the procedure itself (Sasaki G.H. et al., 2014), and for vacuum delivered in pulsed mode (for example, the Z Lipo device by Zimmer, Germany).

Several mechanisms may explain this effect:

- First, mechanical compression of "lipid ice" within adipocytes may further disrupt membranes and organelles, increasing the fraction of cells that die by necrosis or apoptosis.
- Second, massage increases perfusion and oxygen delivery. A sudden increase in oxygen availability can intensify ROS production, disrupt membrane-bound enzymes, and potentially trigger apoptosis via intracellular signaling pathways.

A similar rationale explains why cryolipolysis may become more effective when combined with shockwave therapy. Compared with manual massage, shockwaves deliver higher intensity and penetrate more deeply, reaching deeper SAT layers. They are also more standardized and less dependent on the operator's manual technique (Ferraro G.A. et al., 2012).

5.5. Procedure

A typical cryolipolysis session follows a straightforward sequence (Zelickson B.D. et al., 2015):

1. A gel-impregnated protective pad is placed over the treatment zone. It protects the skin from cold-related injury and helps distribute heat exchange more evenly.
2. The handpiece is positioned over the pad (**Fig. IV-5-14**).
3. After the session, the handpiece and pad are removed, and a post-treatment massage is performed.

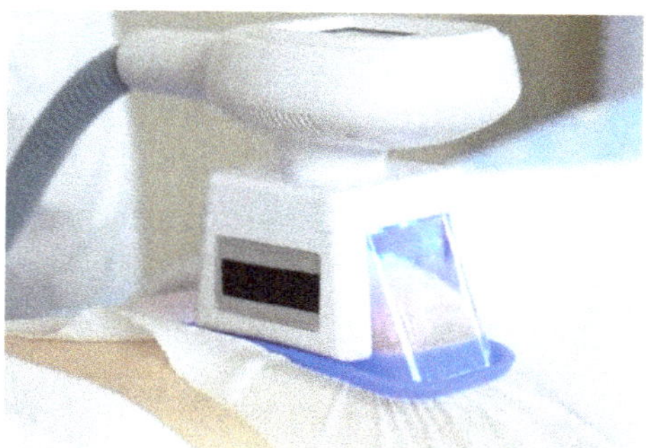

Fig. IV-5-14. Placement of a cryolipolysis handpiece

5.6. Undesirable phenomena and complications

5.6.1. Post-session reactions and complications

Immediately after treatment, the area often appears bright red due to reperfusion. Erythema may persist for several days, reflecting the local inflammatory response. Hematomas and soreness can also last for several days.

Some patients experience temporary skin sensitivity at the contact site with the handpiece. Studies have shown that the density of epidermal nerve fibers decreases in the cooling zone and then gradually — though over a relatively long time — returns toward baseline. Myelinated fibers appear to be affected first, likely because they contain more lipids. These lipids, similar to adipocyte lipids, can crystallize and interfere with nerve conduction (Garibyan L. et al., 2015).

Although cryolipolysis temperatures are not intended to injure the epidermis, dermis, hair follicles, sweat glands, or muscle, frostbite can occur if protocols are violated (for example, incorrect technique or use of uncertified equipment). For safety, cooling plates must not drop below –10 °C. In addition, a dedicated protective gel containing propylene glycol should be used (typically supplied with the manufacturer's pads).

5.6.2. Paradoxical adipose hyperplasia

The first medical report of paradoxical adipose hyperplasia (PAH) appeared in 2014 (Jalian H.R. et al., 2014). By that point, hundreds of thousands of cryolipolysis sessions had already been performed, and 33 cases had been documented, with an estimated incidence of 1 in 20.000 (0.0051%). At the time, both the causes and the predisposing factors were poorly understood, which is why PAH quickly became a focus of active research.

Frequency of occurrence

PAH rates are often reported per procedure or per cycle, which can obscure the real-world risk for the patient who undergoes multiple treatments. Many patients receive several cycles in a single visit (to target different zones) and may repeat sessions over 4–8 weeks. As a result, cumulative PAH risk may be higher than the published cycle-based figures imply. In other words, cycle-by-cycle reporting can underestimate the overall incidence in multi-cycle patients, and this should be explicitly addressed during counseling and consent.

In 2021, the manufacturer of the CoolSculpting system stated a PAH incidence of 0.033% (about 1 case per 3,000 procedures). In contrast, a 2020 systematic review reported an incidence of approximately 0.91% (about 1 case per 110 procedures) — more than 27 times higher than the manufacturer's estimate (Hedayati B. et al., 2020). Some publications have suggested rates as high as 2% (Singh S.M. et al., 2015).

In 2021, a multicenter PAH study analyzed 8,658 cryolipolysis procedures in 2,114 patients (Nikolis A., Enright K.M., 2021). The authors noted that in 76.9% of the PAH cases they reviewed, earlier generations of CoolSculpting systems and handpieces had been used, suggesting a possible technology-related contribution. Older handpieces used two parallel cooling plates and typically ran 60 min per cycle, compared with 35 min for later handpieces with a modified dome shape. The updated dome design sealed more securely to the skin and operated with lower suction force. After these newer handpieces were introduced, PAH cases decreased by 75% even while total procedure volume continued to grow — a strong signal that technical factors matter.

At the time of writing, the most recent cryolipolysis-focused PAH publication is a retrospective review in Aesthetic Surgery (Friedmann D.P. et al., 2025). The authors reviewed electronic medical records of patients treated with commercially available cryolipolysis technology (CoolSculpting and CoolSculpting Elite, Allergan Aesthetics, USA) between January 2016 and June 2023 in a multidisciplinary group practice. Extracted data included the total number of sessions and cycles, cycles and sessions per body region, and treatment-related adverse events. A cycle was defined as one handpiece treating one body area.

The cohort included 3,262 patients (2,797 women and 465 men) who underwent 18,203 cycles across 6,245 sessions. The mean age at the first session was 45 years (range 15–83 years). Mean cycles per patient were 5.6 (median 4). Mean sessions per patient were 1.9 (median 1). The most frequently treated zone was the lower abdomen (N = 1,761; 4,734 cycles), and the most common multi-zone combination was upper/mid + lower abdomen (N = 937; 5,140 cycles). In the subchin region, simultaneous use of two handpieces was more common than a single-handpiece approach. There were 180 adverse events (2.05% of cycles) in 87 patients, including PAH in three body regions (N = 2).

This extensive retrospective review supports the overall safety and broad use of cryolipolysis across multiple anatomical zones. Depending on the calculation method, the per-cycle risk of PAH ranged from 0.018% (1 in 5,501) to 0.048% (1 in 2,063).

Causes

Many aspects of PAH pathophysiology remain unclear. Several mechanisms have been proposed (Jalian H.R. et al., 2014; Stefani W.A., 2015):

- Hypoxic injury
- Hypertrophy of pre-existing adipocytes
- Sympathetic denervation
- Recruitment of preadipocytes
- Changes in receptor expression and/or signaling pathways involved in adipocyte metabolism in response to negative pressure

One hypothesis is that cooling adipocytes without causing enough membrane disruption to kill them may instead push them toward hypertrophy and hyperplasia under hypoxic stress (Stefani W.A., 2015). A commonly cited rationale is that hypoxia can increase the release of hypoxia-inducible factors, which stimulate angiogenesis and may contribute to increased adipocyte size and number (Fong G.H., 2009).

Animal studies also suggest that sympathetic denervation of adipose tissue can suppress lipolysis and increase adipocyte proliferation (Youngstrom T.G., Bartness T.J., 1998; Cousin B. et al., 1993; Hausman D.B. et al., 2001).

Local inflammation may also contribute, via inflammatory cytokines such as tumor necrosis factor-α (TNF-α), which can promote preadipocyte recruitment and potentially support PAH development.

Negative pressure itself has been proposed as a growth stimulus, conceptually similar to tissue expansion effects reported with breast suction devices (Stefani W.A., 2015). However, the magnitude and clinical relevance of this effect in cryolipolysis remain uncertain and require further study.

Another proposed mechanism involves the post-session massage sometimes performed to amplify results. It has been suggested that this massage could cause traumatic injury to adipocyte membranes, leading to inflammatory lipolysis and death of some fat cells through pyroptosis* (Stroumza N. et al., 2018). Pyroptosis resembles apoptosis in that it is programmed, but it is distinctly inflammatory. In this model, inflammatory lipolysis is caspase-1-dependent and involves membrane pore formation, disruption of ion gradients, and osmotic cell swelling. Cytokines, including pro-inflammatory mediators, are released through these pores. If the cell cannot reseal the membrane in time, the process becomes irreversible and the cell-death program proceeds (Bergsbaken T. et al., 2009).

The literature is not entirely consistent regarding structural changes in adipose tissue after cryolipolysis in PAH. For example, Seaman S.A. et al. (2016) followed patients for 7 months post-treatment and described reduced vascularization and fewer living interstitial cells (including macrophages, endothelial cells, adipose-derived stem cells, and blood cells) involved in adipose remodeling (**Fig. IV-5-15**). Jalian H.R. et al. (2014) reported the opposite pattern — increased vascular and capillary density in the fat layer of a PAH patient at 3 months post-treatment.

---

* Pyroptosis is a programmed necrotic form of cell death in which caspase-1 activation disrupts plasma-membrane integrity and cellular contents are rapidly released outward. Pyroptosis is characterized by caspase-1-dependent release of interleukins IL-1β and IL-18, which drive inflammation. It functions as a protective mechanism of innate immunity that limits intracellular pathogen replication, but it is not limited to bacterial infections (Wikipedia).

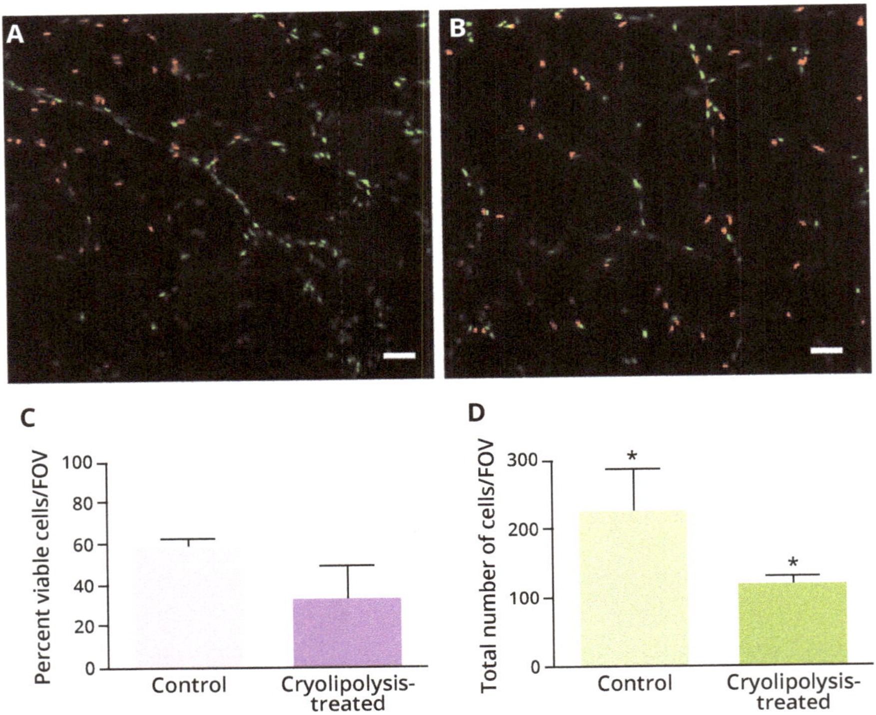

Fig. IV-5-15. Decrease in percentage of viable interstitial cells and total interstitial cells in cryolipolysis-treated tissue compared to control tissue (adapted from Seaman S.A. et al., 2016; CC BY)

Tissue samples from (A) control and (B) cryolipolysis-treated tissue were stained using the LIVE/DEAD kit to assess (C) interstitial cell viability and (D) total interstitial cell counts. Representative images and quantification of three fields of view show a lower percentage of viable cells in cryolipolysis-treated tissue compared to control tissue (B) and a statistically significant decrease in the total number of interstitial cells in cryolipolysis-treated tissue (D). To assess statistical significance ($P < 0.05$), a two-sided paired t-test was used for both quantification methods. Scale bar = 50 μm.

Risk factors

The following PAH risk factors have been described (Kelly E. et al., 2016; Nikolis A., Enright K.M., 2021):

- **Male patients:** although men account for only about 15% of cryolipolysis procedures, roughly half of reported PAH cases occur in this group
- **Abdominal region:** treatment of the abdomen is associated with a higher risk

- **Extensive handpiece use:** handpiece size may influence risk
- **Repeated cryolipolysis:** higher treatment frequency may contribute
- **Genetic characteristics:** PAH has been reported in male twins and may be more common among individuals of Hispanic descent
- **Technical factors:** PAH is reported more often with older handpieces using two parallel cooling plates with 60-minute cycles, compared with newer contoured, dome-shaped handpieces using 35-min cycles and lower suction force

Some authors have suggested that shockwave therapy may have a protective effect against PAH. For example, Michon A. (2021) reported that over nearly 4 years of clinical practice, 2,291 cryolipolysis procedures followed by shockwave therapy were performed at the author's clinic, with no cases of PAH observed during that period. The author proposed that the mechanical, anti-inflammatory, and circulation-supporting effects of shockwave therapy may improve cryolipolysis outcomes and reduce the risk of adverse events, including PAH. They also noted less edema and discomfort in patients who received shockwave therapy in combination with cryolipolysis.

Chapter 6
Combined technologies

Individual sensitivity is a central issue in any energy-based exposure. For some people, treatment produces the desired response; for others, it triggers unwanted reactions. That is why the clinician has to balance efficacy against the risk of side effects. One practical strategy is to combine different modalities at doses that do not injure tissue.

According to the Arndt–Schultz rule, the dose-response curve for physiologic effects has a parabolic shape (**Fig. IV-6-1**): "Small doses of drugs stimulate, medium doses enhance, large doses depress, and huge doses paralyze the activity of living elements." Although this rule was formulated for pharmaceuticals, it has since been shown that physical exposures follow a similar pattern.

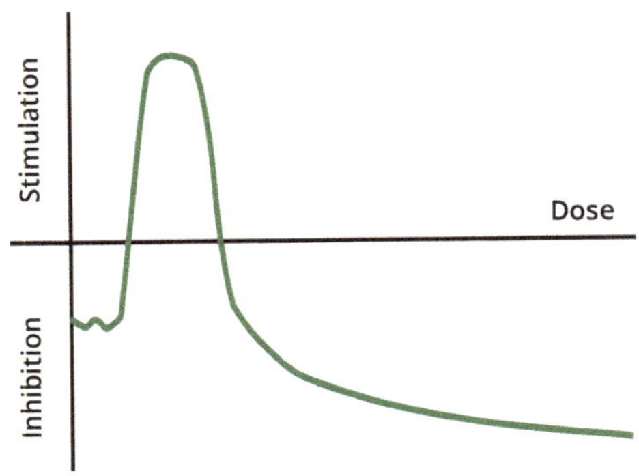

Fig. IV-6-1. Arndt–Schultz rule

Many recent innovations center on combining multiple physical modalities. This is not just about sequencing different methods across a course. Increasingly, two or more factors are delivered simultaneously or in a tightly integrated way within a single session via a single platform. Many such platforms are available today, and some were already mentioned in earlier chapters. A few additional examples are outlined below.

One of the earliest combined approaches to become widely adopted in aesthetic practice is ELOS technology, developed by Syneron (Israel). The name reflects two modalities: alternating electric current in the radiofrequency range (electrical effect) and electromagnetic waves in the light range (optical effect). In a well-balanced pairing, these two factors support natural skin regeneration and contribute to structural rejuvenation.

Modern platforms may combine more than two modalities. For example, the VelaShape platform (Syneron, Israel), designed for cellulite management, uses four physical factors: IR radiation, RF current, vacuum aspiration, and roller massage. This combination helps address multiple pathogenic links involved in cellulite formation. Rotating rollers redistribute interstitial fluid toward lymphatic pathways, easing bottlenecks in lymphatic and venous outflow. Improved microcirculation and drainage are especially helpful in early-stage cellulite. Later, thicker fibrous septa form around adipocytes, restricting metabolic exchange. The challenge grows because, as aging and cellulite progress, additional cross-links form in fibrillar proteins, increasing resistance to proteolytic enzymes. These "aged" proteins accumulate in the extracellular matrix and become harder to clear. Heating the dermis with RF promotes denaturation of "old" collagen, accelerating its breakdown and subsequent replacement with newly formed fibers. IR also warms the skin, acting mainly in the more superficial layers and helping reduce inflammatory activity.

Among combined technologies, the Multi Polar Magnetic Pulse $(MP)^2$ approach (Venus Concept, Israel) pairs multipolar RF with pulsed electromagnetic fields. Together, these factors support structural improvement in dermal collagen fibers, stimulate circulation in SAT, enhance nutrient and oxygen delivery, and promote lipolysis.

Simultaneous exposure to several physical factors is not always possible or necessary. Still, it is convenient to have multiple options available within the same program. For this reason, multifunctional platforms are built with several handpieces that operate across different modalities. For example, the Lumicell Wave 7 platform (Silhouet-Tone, Canada) includes four handpieces used at various stages of a treatment plan.

Treatment intensity is adjusted individually, based on the stage of cellulite and the volume of fat deposits:

1. The session commonly begins with rhythmic photopneumatic massage: vacuum-roller kneading of subcutaneous fatty tissue

helps soften fibrous structures, reduce lymph stagnation, and improve circulation. At the same time, IR light produces deep heating (up to 5 cm, up to 40 °C), which can support lipid release from adipocytes (via effects on β-adrenoreceptors), provide a biostimulating influence, improve trophic support, and stimulate new collagen production.
2. Active lipolytic components are delivered transdermally using electroporation.
3. Ultrasonic thermolipolysis is applied. High-frequency cavitation increases adipocyte membrane permeability and disrupts the organization of fibrous septa. The heat generated also stimulates catecholamine production, which, in turn, activates lipolysis.
4. Integrated RF therapy increases skin density through diathermy.

When several modalities are combined within a single procedure and applied at different stages, their effects accumulate, often producing a brighter, longer-lasting outcome than any single method alone. In addition, this approach is frequently safer because each modality can be used at a lower intensity, with overall efficacy maintained through complementary action.

Part V

Injection treatment

Mesotherapy is an injection-based technique in which biologically active substances are introduced into the skin. It is widely used to improve the condition and appearance of skin and hair. Meso solutions may contain one active ingredient or several. Multi-ingredient formulations are often called "meso cocktails". A meso cocktail may be sold as a ready-to-use product or prepared by mixing components immediately before injection. **The key requirement is compatibility: combined ingredients should be physically, chemically, and pharmacologically compatible.** In addition to formulated mixtures, mesotherapy also uses animal- or plant-derived extracts — complex blends of water-soluble substances.

Using mesotherapy to stimulate lipolysis is supported by clinical experience and observations, suggesting that intradermal delivery of meso solutions can reduce the volume of fat depots. Recall that cellulite development involves four main pathogenetic processes: (1) microcirculatory impairment with local tissue hypoxia, (2) adipocyte hypertrophy, (3) inflammation, and (4) fibrosis. With mesotherapy, it is possible to influence each of these.

1.1. Improvement of microcirculation

At any stage of cellulite, restoring adequate drainage through the circulatory and lymphatic systems is essential so that adipose-tissue breakdown products can be cleared without delay.

Ingredients used to strengthen the vascular wall, reduce capillary permeability, and support circulation include:

1. Vitamins K, E, C, H
2. Rutin
3. Organic silicon

4. Mesoglycan
5. Buflomedil (Loftyl)
6. Extracts of fucus, ginkgo, melilotus (meliloto), and artichoke

Meso solutions are administered using classic capillary-vascular mesotherapy patterns, following the main vascular pathways and the spinal column.

A vascular session may be performed as a standalone treatment or scheduled before adipose-tissue targeting. Combining vascular-active agents with lipolytics is also an option.

When multiple products are used in the same visit, they are injected at different skin depths using separate syringes. That said, a more cautious and often preferable approach is to separate vascular-active sessions and lipolytic sessions by a few days.

1.2. Impact on adipose tissue

Effects on SAT volume can be grouped into two broad directions:

1. **Without adipocyte destruction** (physiologic regulation of lipolysis):
   - Stimulation of triglyceride breakdown
   - Reduction of triglyceride synthesis
2. **With adipocyte destruction** (lipodestruction):
   - Emulsification of fat ("fat dissolution")
   - Osmotic destruction (osmotic shock)
   - Cryodestruction

1.2.1. Physiologic regulation of lipolysis

Reducing lipid stores within adipocytes can be approached in two ways. The first is stimulating lipolysis — activating triglyceride breakdown. Substances used for this purpose are commonly called **lipolysis activators**. The second is reducing lipogenesis — decreasing the adipocyte's capacity to synthesize and store triglycerides. Substances used for this purpose are called **lipogenesis inhibitors**.

Unlike lipodestructors (see below), lipolysis activators do not eliminate fat cells. As a result, their effect is typically less dramatic and more temporary: "slimmed down" adipocytes can regain volume over time.

At the same time, lipolysis activators offer practical advantages:

- Their mechanism is more physiologic, because it works through the body's native fat-metabolism pathways.
- They can be used across a larger body surface area and in larger total volumes than lipodestructors.
- They tend to have fewer restrictions and contraindications.

Three enzymes participate in lipolysis: triglyceride lipase (TGL), diglyceride lipase (DGL), and monoglyceride lipase (MGL). The activity of DGL and MGL is 10–100 times higher than that of TGL. However, TGL is the rate-limiting step and effectively "sets the speed" of the process (**Fig. V-1**).

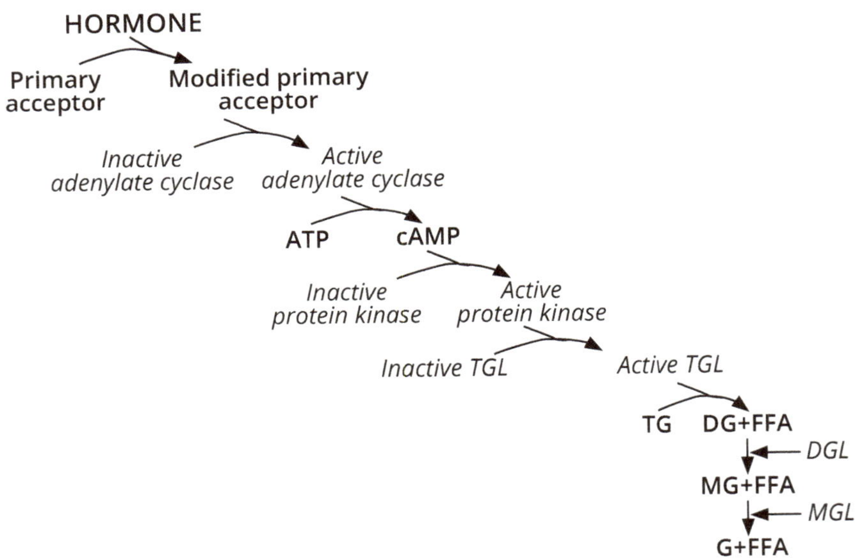

Fig. V-1. Lipolytic cascade in adipocytes (adapted from Steinberg D., 1972; CC BY)

Abbreviations: G — glycerol; MG — monoglyceride; DG — diglyceride; TG — triglyceride; FFA — free fatty acid; MGL — monoglyceride lipase; DGL — diglyceride lipase; TGL — triglyceride lipase

The lipolytic cascade proceeds through a sequence of steps:

1. It begins when a hormone binds to the β-adrenergic receptor on the adipocyte membrane, changing the receptor's structure (the hormone itself does not enter the cell).
2. The modified receptor activates adenylate cyclase, which catalyzes the formation of cyclic adenosine monophosphate (cAMP) from adenosine triphosphate (ATP).
3. cAMP activates protein kinase A, which phosphorylates TGL, converting it to its active form.
4. Activated TGL cleaves triglycerides into diglycerides and fatty acids.
5. Then, through the sequential action of DGL and MGL, the end products of lipolysis — glycerol and free fatty acids — are produced and released into the blood.

In complex with plasma albumin, fatty acids are transported via the blood to organs and tissues, where the complex dissociates. Fatty acids are then either β-oxidized or used (in part) to synthesize triglycerides, glycerophospholipids, sphingophospholipids, and other compounds, and they also participate in cholesterol esterification.

The rate of triglyceride cleavage is not constant. It is shaped by multiple regulatory inputs (**Table V-1**), with neurohormonal signals playing a vital role. TGL is activated by hormones such as adrenaline, noradrenaline, and glucagon, which is why it is also called hormone-sensitive lipase. In contrast, DGL and MGL are not regulated by these hormones (**Fig. V-2**).

A key intracellular regulator of lipolysis is cAMP. Its concentration depends on the balance between two enzymes with opposing actions: adenylate cyclase (cAMP synthesis) and phosphodiesterase (cAMP breakdown). By influencing these enzymes, lipolysis can be modulated.

Among mesotherapy lipolysis activators, different mechanisms are represented. For example:

- Artichoke extract can increase adenylate cyclase activity, raising intracellular cAMP.
- Caffeine can produce a similar rise by inhibiting phosphodiesterase, slowing cAMP breakdown.

Table V-1. Effect of selected factors on triglyceride breakdown in adipose tissue

FACTOR	RESULT	PUTATIVE MECHANISM OF ACTION
Catecholamines Glucagon Thyroxine Glucocorticoids Growth hormone Adrenocortico-tropic hormone	Enhancement	Adenylate cyclase activation
Stress Physical activity Starvation Cooling	Amplification	• Increase in catecholamine secretion • Decrease in insulin secretion
Insulin	Suppression	• Phosphodiesterase activation (increased cAMP hydrolysis) • Decrease in adenylate cyclase activity
Prostaglandins Nicotinic acid	Suppression	• Decrease in adenylate cyclase activity

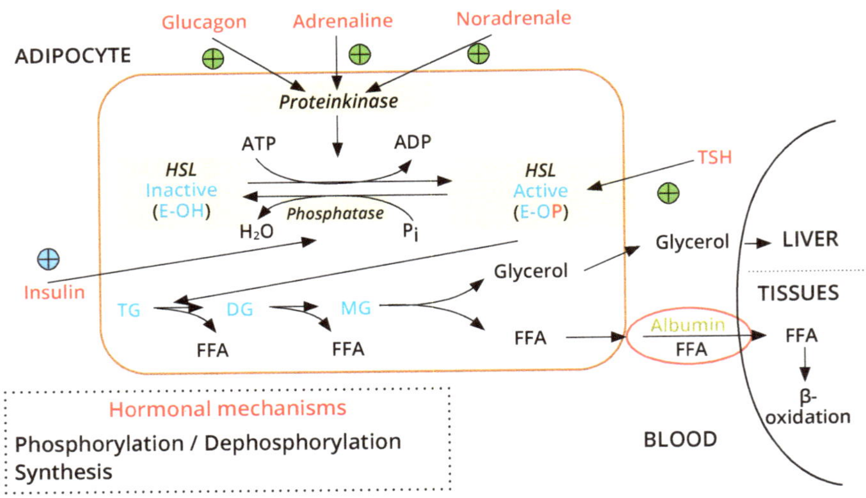

Fig. V-2. Hormonal regulation of lipolysis in adipocytes

Abbreviations: TSH — somatotropic hormone; FFA — free fatty acids; HSL — hormone-sensitive lipase; P_i — inorganic phosphate; TG — triglyceride; DG — diglyceride; MG — monoglyceride

- Organic silicon and centella extract are also described as supporting higher intracellular cAMP.
- Some components additionally support triglyceride breakdown into di- and monoglycerides.
- L-carnitine facilitates the transport of mono- and diglycerides and fatty acids into mitochondria for subsequent utilization.

The importance of selecting compatible, functionally coherent combinations is illustrated by Caruso M.K. et al. (2008), who compared the lipolytic activity of different compositions in a human fat-cell culture model. Lipolysis efficiency was assessed by measuring glycerol release. The following solutions were tested:

- Aminophylline
- Yohimbine
- Isoproterenol
- Meliloto
- Aminophylline + meliloto
- Aminophylline + isoproterenol
- Aminophylline + isoproterenol + yohimbine
- Aminophylline + isoproterenol + lidocaine
- Aminophylline + isoproterenol + yohimbine + lidocaine

A buffer solution served as the control. Lipolytic activity of isoproterenol ($P < 0.002$), aminophylline ($P < 0.00004$), and yohimbine ($P < 0.001$) was significantly higher than that of the control (**Fig. V-3**). Lipolysis stimulation induced by meliloto ($P < 0.01$) and isoproterenol ($P < 0.002$) increased when aminophylline was added ($P < 0.001$ and $P < 0.001$, respectively). At the same time, the stimulation produced by aminophylline + isoproterenol ($P < 0.0009$) and by aminophylline + isoproterenol + yohimbine ($P < 0.0007$) was inhibited by lidocaine. Even with lidocaine present, the aminophylline + isoproterenol + yohimbine combination still induced lipolysis more strongly than control ($P < 0.05$) (Caruso M.K. et al., 2008).

Practically, this study supports two takeaways:

- First, several commonly used mesotherapy ingredients can stimulate lipolysis on their own, and in combination, they may enhance one another.

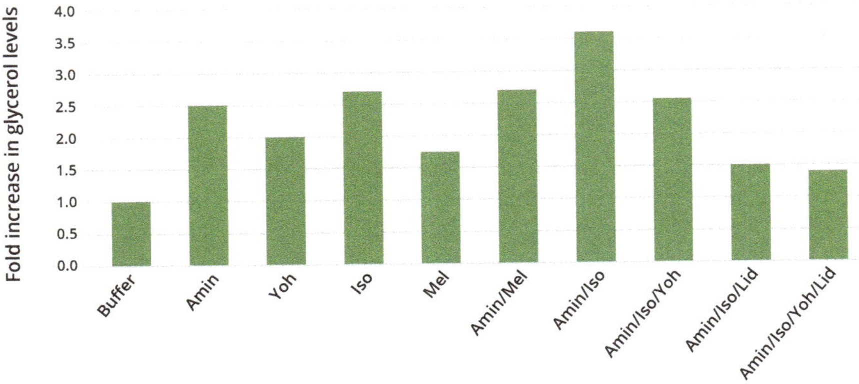

Fig. V-3. Comparative lipolytic activity of the tested solutions compared to buffer (adapted from Caruso M.K. et al., 2008; CC BY)

Abbreviations: Amin — aminophylline; Yoh — yohimbine; Iso, isoproterenol; Mel — meliloto (turfgrass extract); Amin/Mel — aminophylline + meliloto; Amin/Iso — aminophylline + isoproterenol; Amin/Iso/ioh — aminophylline + isoproterenol + yohimbine; Amin/Iso/Lid — aminophylline + isoproterenol + lidocaine; Amin/Iso/Yoh/Lid — aminophylline + isoproterenol + yohimbine + lidocaine

- Second — and clinically meaningful — local anesthetics can inhibit lipolysis. The authors' conclusion is direct: anesthetics should be excluded from meso cocktails intended to address cellulite and localized fat deposits.

1.2.2. Lipodestruction

Adipocyte destruction can be achieved in several ways: emulsification driven by surfactants, osmotic swelling followed by rupture after injection of a hypotonic solution, and cooling using injected ice microfragments.

Fat emulsification ("fat dissolution")

Emulsification is the process of combining two immiscible liquids (for example, oil and water) into a uniform, stable mixture called an emulsion. Mechanical forces (vigorous shaking, stirring, ultrasonication) break one liquid into tiny droplets that disperse throughout the other. Those droplets are coated with an emulsifier layer that prevents coalescence and helps keep the emulsion stable. In other words, an emulsifier is the third essential component of an emulsion.

An emulsifier has an affinity for both water and oil. In an emulsion, it sits at the interface between the two phases — on the droplet surface — which places it in the surfactant class. Surfactants are used not only to create emulsions, but also broadly in soaps and detergents because they can generate foam and help remove hydrophobic contaminants, including grease. They integrate into fatty deposits, loosen them, and weaken their attachment to surfaces, making them easier to wash away.

In the body, abnormal lipid deposits can develop under certain conditions — for example, plaques on the inner vessel wall in atherosclerosis, or lipid accumulation in the liver in steatohepatosis ("fatty liver"). Intravenous formulations based on surfactants that are closely related to endogenous molecules — phosphatidylcholine (PC; also known as lecithin) and sodium deoxycholate (DC) — are also used as part of combined therapy in these conditions (**Fig. V-4**). This approach is referred to as injectable lipolysis, and under that name it also became established in aesthetic practice as a subcutaneous injection technique.

The aesthetic use of injectable lipolysis traces back to 1959, when an early report described a successful attempt to dissolve a fat embolus using lecithin. The following report on a similar theme appeared only in 1988: Sergio Maggiore used an injectable form of PC for local treatment of xanthelasma — lipid deposits that most often occur on eyelid skin and are associated with lipid-metabolism disorders. In 1995, Brazilian physician Patricia Rittes reported successful correction of lower-eyelid fat herniation using subcutaneous PC injections. That publication drew the attention of plastic surgeons and opened a new direction in aesthetic medicine.

In many European countries, several **intravenously administered** PC-containing medications are registered and manufactured by pharmaceutical companies under pharmaceutical production standards. For example (per a drug reference source):

- Lipostabil (Aventis, Germany): PC 5%, DC 2.5%
- Essentiale N (A. Nattermann & Cie GmbH, Germany): PC 5%, DC 2.5%

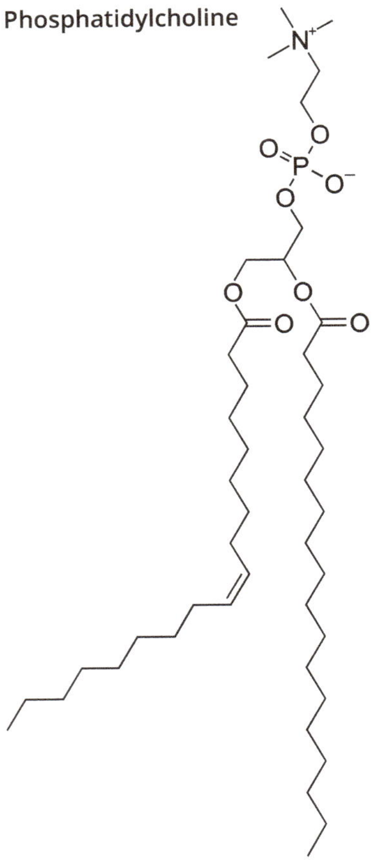

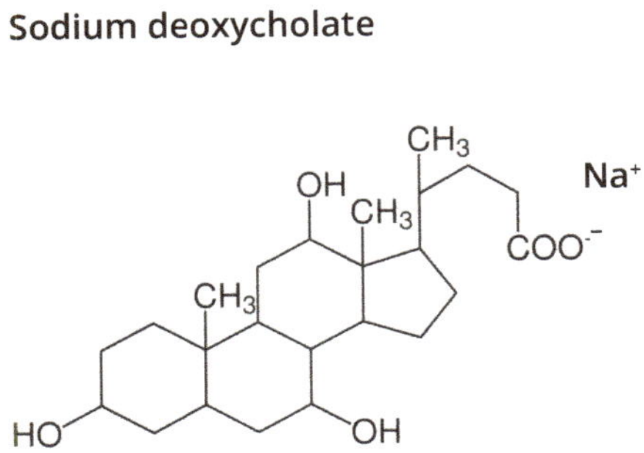

Fig. V-4. Structural formulas of natural surfactants — components of injectable solutions for dissolving localized fat deposits

There are also products marketed for aesthetic injectable lipolysis via **subcutaneous administration**, produced by cosmetic manufacturers. For example (per manufacturers' websites):

- Dermastabilon (Skin Rebirth, Spain): PC 5%, DC 2%
- INNO-TDS Draining PPC (Innosearch, Spain): PC 5%
- F-PPC (Oxynergy Paris Group, Spain): PC 5%, DC 2.5%

It is important to emphasize that **using registered intravenously administered medications as subcutaneous injections for localized fat reduction is off-label**. As for cosmetic products, they do not undergo the same required preclinical and clinical testing pathway.

A special mention should be made of Kybella/Belkyra (Kythera Biopharmaceuticals/Allergan, USA), which is administered by subcutaneous injection into the submental area to reduce the appearance of a "double chin." The product was introduced in the U.S. and Canada in 2017 and in Europe in 2017. Kybella is currently the only FDA-approved medication in this category. It contains a single active ingredient: 1% DC.

Aesthetic injectable lipolysis is an intensive intervention: the drug is placed directly into fat to induce relatively rapid adipocyte destruction. In this context, the classic mesotherapy concept — using small doses to create a local depot within the skin — does not really apply. For that reason, many experts argue that correcting localized fat deposits with surfactants should not be labeled as mesotherapy (Rotunda A.M., Kolodney M.S., 2006).

In most injectable "fat reducers", the principal active ingredient is PC, a major lipid component of cell membranes. The proportion of PC among total membrane lipids varies by cell type and also by where the membrane sits within the cell: the lowest PC content is found in the plasma membrane (about 20% w/w), while the highest is in endoplasmic reticulum membranes (up to 50% w/w). Membrane integrity depends on a balanced lipid composition, and a marked shift in that balance can lead to structural disruption — or even membrane failure. PC readily incorporates into membranes. Once a critical local concentration is reached, the membrane can rupture, releasing cellular contents — including lipid droplets — into the extracellular space. PC can also integrate into those droplets and fragment them into smaller ones, which are then cleared.

Early work on injectable lipolysis largely extrapolated the pharmacologic effects of IV PC (observed in serum) directly to adipose tissue. Later cell-culture experiments showed that achieving effective adipocyte membrane destruction with PC alone required concentrations deemed unsafe. That pushed researchers toward a "partner" ingredient that could facilitate membrane lysis and improve PC access to lipid droplets. Sodium deoxycholate (DC), the sodium salt of deoxycholic acid, was selected for this role (Rotunda A.M. et al., 2004; Salti G. et al., 2008). Deoxycholic acid is a bile acid and is structurally related to endogenous compounds.

In the "DC + PC" pairing, DC is generally viewed as the component that disrupts membrane permeability and drives adipocyte lysis, leading to the release of intracellular contents into the extracellular space — that is, tissue necrosis. PC is then thought to emulsify extracellular triglycerides, forming lipid droplets that are later phagocytosed by macrophages and multinucleated giant cells (Duncan D.I., Hasengschwandtner F., 2005; Rose P.T., Morgan M., 2005). The appearance of nodular infiltrates after injection supports the idea that inflammation — an intrinsic part of necrosis — can ultimately lead to fibrosis. Cellular debris is then cleared by macrophages, transported systemically via the lymphatic system, and metabolized in the liver (Duncan D.I. et al., 2009).

Treatments are typically scheduled every 2–8 weeks. Longer intervals (up to 8 weeks) are often recommended because they allow inflammation to resolve fully and SAT remodeling to begin. By about the third month, skin retraction is generally complete. Results can persist for a long time as long as body weight remains stable.

Expected immediate post-injection reactions include swelling, erythema, itching, and/or burning. Ecchymoses and edema may persist for several days and, in some cases, for weeks. These effects reflect localized inflammation and necrosis within SAT and usually resolve spontaneously. The inflammatory phase commonly lasts from a few hours to 10 days, although persistent macrophage activity lasting up to 3 weeks has been reported. Moderately painful nodules may remain for roughly a month after treatment.

The most common drivers of complications are technique errors and the use of uncertified products (Kaur H. et al., 2022). Injections that are too deep or too superficial can cause necrosis of muscle or skin, regardless of concentration. Breaks in asepsis and antisepsis increase the risk of infection. Allergic reactions also matter: PC is typically soy-derived, so patients should be asked specifically about soy allergy.

To reduce the risk of overdosing and overly tight injection spacing, the Kybella/Belkyra protocol uses a standardized marking system: a grid-like template is applied, and 0.2 ml aliquots are injected into pre-marked points at 1 cm intervals (Fagien S. et al., 2016).

Aesthetic injectable lipolysis will not replace liposuction, but it may compete with technology-based approaches in selected cases. Today, PC/DC injectables are mainly used to reduce small, localized subcutaneous fat pads that do not respond well to diet and exercise.

When clinicians analyzed failures in cellulite management with PC and DC, it became clear that simply "dissolving fat" via injection is rarely enough for a good outcome. A comprehensive plan is needed — one that accounts for the etiology and pathophysiology of gynoid lipodystrophy and supports both the vascular component and connective-tissue architecture.

A lack of clear methodological guidance sometimes leads clinicians — especially when results disappoint, or complications occur — to take on avoidable risks: increasing doses beyond accepted safety limits, lowering doses below effective ranges, or mixing PC/DC formulations with mesotherapy agents. These choices can alter physicochemical and biological behavior, leading to unpredictable outcomes.

Indications:

- Small fat deposits (up to 500 ml)
- Residual fat deposits after liposuction
- Excess fat volume after fat grafting
- Selected lipomas (single lipomas are generally better managed surgically)

Contraindications and precautions (Mahmud K., Crutchfield C.E., 2012):

- Avoid use in pregnant patients and in patients with systemic conditions such as cardiac or renal disease, uncontrolled diabetes, uncompensated hypothyroidism, infections, active or past autoimmune disease, or active skin lesions.
- Avoid use in patients taking aspirin or other anti-inflammatory drugs, and in those with increased bleeding tendency.
- Avoid use in individuals with soy allergy, because the standard PC/DC blend is soy-derived.
- Do not inject in the breast or axillary region to avoid potentially stimulating malignant-cell development.

- Avoid injecting near the knees (close to ligaments) or below the knee, as these areas are more vulnerable to skin injury.
- Use the minimum adequate volume needed for the specific zone and fat volume, typically 40–60 ml.
- Place injections 1.5 cm apart, centered within the fat pad, avoiding the skin, muscle, and fascia.
- Avoid rubbing the treated area and avoid tight clothing.
- After treatment, avoid applying lotions to reduce the risk of infection and allow the puncture sites to heal for a few days.

Procedure recommendations (Mahmud K., Crutchfield C.E., 2012):

- **Patient selection:** Choose patients with well-localized, soft fat pads; avoid dense, fibrotic deposits, which tend to respond poorly.
- **Injection technique:** In patients with cellulite or skin laxity, injections may be placed slightly more superficially, but still at least 5 mm deep, while avoiding areas with marked laxity and minimal fat thickness.
- **Pre-procedure assessment:** Palpate carefully and mark accurately, accounting for individual anatomy (for example, a fat roll around the umbilicus, larger zones above or below the umbilicus, and multiple abdominal regions).
- **Ultrasound use:** To enhance the effect, ultrasound may be used before or immediately after treatment to promote adipocyte destruction.
- **Injection interval:** To optimize the initial result, wait 6–8 weeks before treating the same area again.

Hypotonic destruction of adipocytes

A different lipodestruction approach involves injecting a hypotonic solution*. This method was introduced by American plastic surgeon Steve Hoefflin in 1999 and described as **hypotonic pharmacologic lipodissolution** (Hoefflin S.M., 1999, 2002). It relies on osmosis — the spontaneous movement of solvent (here, water) from a lower-osmolarity environment (the extracellular space) into a higher-osmolarity

---

* Hypotonic solution is a solution where the concentration of dissolved substances is lower than in the cell.

medium (the cell) across a semipermeable membrane (the cell membrane). When a hypotonic solution is injected into SAT, adipocytes swell and may rupture, disrupting the localized fat deposit (Park S.Y. et al., 2024). Even in refined versions used in some surgical practices, this method has not become widely adopted.

Injectable cryolipolysis

The first publication on injectable cryolipolysis appeared in 2020 (Garibyan L. et al., 2020). The concept itself is not new — invasive cryoprobes have been used for years to ablate neoplasms and other pathologic tissues. The problem is selectivity: classic cryoprobes cool tissue to subzero temperatures, which is not ideal when you want to target adipocytes while sparing surrounding structures preferentially.

To address this, a special formulation was developed: a suspension of small ice particles in a liquid carrier. The heat absorbed by this suspension during melting is roughly 80 times greater than the heat capacity of water. By injecting an ice suspension, you can cool the target tissue directly without overcooling the skin's more superficial layers.

Initial testing was performed in Yorkshire pigs (Garibyan L. et al., 2020). Injectable suspensions were prepared using physiologic solution and glycerol in different ratios to create mixtures containing 20% and 40% ice (the final experimental version included 10% glycerol). Glycerol lowers the freezing point of the mix, allowing it to remain injectable even below 0 °C: in mixtures containing 20% and 40% ice, the freezing points were –3.5 °C and –4.8 °C, respectively. Injections were performed under general anesthesia directly into SAT to a depth of about 2 cm using a 15G needle, with 30 ml injected. Ultrasound and histologic assessments were performed at baseline and at 8 weeks post-treatment, and the animals were photographed.

Ultrasound imaging immediately after injection showed a hyperechogenic rim with acoustic shadowing — consistent with strong acoustic reflection from ice particles. A few minutes later, the hyperechogenic rim expanded in diameter, suggesting lipid crystallization within the adipose tissue. As lipid crystals and ice particles melted, the hyperechogenic zone gradually diminished and then disappeared.

At 8 weeks, subcutaneous fat thickness in the injected area decreased by 27.7 ± 4.6% versus baseline. In animals injected with the control solution, average fat-layer thickness increased by 52.1 ± 8.8% over the same period, reflecting normal growth during the study. The magnitude of effect depended on both suspension temperature and injected volume — lower temperatures and larger volumes produced stronger results.

Histology showed that the treated area initially contained no inflammatory cells and was composed of 97% adipose tissue. By day 3 after injection, mild diffuse inflammation around fat lobules was observed. Inflammation peaked between 14 and 28 days, when dense lymphocytic infiltrates (including multinucleated giant cells/macrophages) and features of lobular panniculitis were documented. A substantial number of lipid-laden macrophages were present by day 14, consistent with active phagocytosis. In the injection zones, adipose thickness decreased, while fibrous septa in the remaining adipose tissue became thicker (reflected by higher collagen-fiber density) and more cellular. The number of myofibroblasts within septa also increased. None of these findings were observed at control injection sites. Significantly, the observed effects were limited to adipose tissue. No damage to the epidermis, dermis, skin appendages (including hair follicles and sweat glands), or muscle tissue was detected at any point in the study.

Laboratory monitoring (blood chemistry, liver function, lipid profile) at baseline, on day 3, and at 2-, 4-, and 8-week follow-up did not reveal abnormalities. Overall, these processes align with the descriptions of classic cryolipolysis.

At 4 weeks after injection, visible skin indentations were noted, reflecting selective loss of subcutaneous fat. By week 8, these indentations enlarged. Control sites injected with a similar formulation containing melted ice did not show indentations.

Clinically, mild swelling and erythema appeared within 10–15 min after injection. No infection, ulceration, pigment changes, scarring, tissue necrosis, or systemic side effects were seen during observation. There were no reports of unexpected animal behavior suggestive of pain or distress.

The first human study was published in 2021 (Kandula P. et al., 2021). It enrolled patients scheduled for abdominoplasty. Before surgery (and during follow-up), an ice suspension was injected directly into the SAT in areas that were later excised. In the control group, a melted ice suspension was infiltrated into the same zones.

Results showed that a single injection could lower adipose-tissue temperature below the target of 10 °C. No serious adverse events were reported; the most common were hematoma and erythema. Average discomfort (10-point scale) was low: 1.9 in ice-suspension sites and 1.3 in control sites.

Instrument-based assessments — thermography, ultrasound, and histology — confirmed that ice-suspension injection produces localized cooling and induces cryolipolysis specifically at injection sites, without meaningful changes in control areas.

Overall, early evidence suggests that injectable cryolipolysis has a favorable safety and tolerability profile and can effectively cool adipose tissue, supporting selective adipocyte destruction. It also looks promising as a more precise and adaptable approach to subcutaneous fat, though further studies are needed to optimize it and facilitate broader clinical adoption.

1.3. Skin thickening

1.3.1. Mesotherapy

A necessary part of anti-cellulite therapy — especially during active lipolytic work and reduction of fat deposits — is improving skin density, elasticity, and turgor.

The most common meso-solution components used for this purpose are ingredients that support the synthesis of new extracellular-matrix components:

- Hyaluronic acid (native)
- Dimethylaminoethanol (DMAE)
- Organic silicon (monomethyl trisilanol salicylate)
- Lipoic acid
- Amino acids
- Nucleotides

These products are administered intradermally using multipuncture, linear, or papular techniques. Across the treatment course, it is recommended to alternate skin-tone support sessions with lipolytic sessions.

1.3.2. Collagen therapy

In recent years, collagen therapy has become increasingly popular. This technique involves injecting collagen-based preparations directly into the dermis. Injectable collagen used in cosmetic procedures is most commonly derived from animal skin — primarily cattle and pigs — with a preference for young cattle.

Producing injectable collagen begins with extracting collagen from animal skin, a complex and costly step due to limited raw material availability and stringent safety and quality requirements. This is followed by careful purification to remove impurities and potential allergens. In some cases, deamination is performed to modify collagen structure and improve water retention in the skin. Standardization is essential to maintaining consistent product properties from batch to batch. Raw materials are tested for virologic and microbiologic safety to reduce infection risk.

The finished product may be supplied as a ready-to-use gel or as a powder that requires pre-hydration. Quality control is applied throughout manufacturing, from supplier selection to ensuring maximal purity of all reagents (Ni H. et al., 2023). In parallel, recombinant collagen produced biotechnologically using microorganisms is emerging as an alternative to animal-derived collagen. Early reports of successful trials with injectable recombinant collagen III for age-related changes have already been published (Tao L., Yi Y., 2025).

Immediately after treatment, the skin often appears visibly thicker, although this early effect is temporary. Injected collagen is partially fragmented during manufacturing and is rapidly broken down by collagenases. This breakdown releases matrikines (signal peptides) that stimulate fibroblasts to synthesize endogenous collagen. As the dermal matrix reorganizes, the skin becomes denser, pores appear smaller, the capillary network becomes less visually prominent, and overall skin quality improves. Unlike hyaluronic acid products, collagen preparations do not attract water or increase tissue volume.

Collagen is injected into the dermis using a micropapular technique to help evenly distribute it throughout the tissue. A typical initial course includes 3–5 sessions at roughly 3–4-week intervals, followed by maintenance treatments every 3–4 months.

Indications:

- Consequences of significant weight loss (excess skin) and liposuction
- Age-related skin changes (wrinkles, reduced elasticity, sagging)
- Scars and stretch marks
- Skin preparation for other aesthetic procedures and recovery afterward
- Comprehensive therapy for the prevention and correction of age-related changes

Contraindications:

- Skin diseases in an exacerbation phase
- Infectious diseases
- Chronic vascular pathology
- Chronic renal failure, nephropathy
- Pregnancy, lactation
- Acute febrile diseases
- Blood coagulation disorders
- Epilepsy
- Tendency toward keloid-scar formation
- Individual intolerance
- Allergy history: relative contraindication, requires allergy testing

1.4. Carboxytherapy

RIn recent years, many aesthetic clinics have increasingly offered carboxytherapy as another option for addressing cellulite.

Historically, the medical use of carbon dioxide is firmly rooted in balneology. Dry CO_2 baths were recognized back in the 19th century. Later, their therapeutic effects across a broad range of conditions were confirmed clinically and experimentally, and today they are used in cardiology, pulmonology, orthopedics, rheumatology, dermatology, and sports medicine.

Today, the term "carboxytherapy" most often refers to a specific technique: subcutaneous injection of CO_2, although non-invasive CO_2 delivery methods are sometimes included under the same label.

In the literature, you may also see the term "pneumopuncture" — intradermal injection of CO_2 into acupuncture points that are reflexively linked to the affected organ.

Although carboxytherapy is often presented as an innovation in aesthetic medicine, its history in clinical practice goes back to 1932 in France, where intradermal and subcutaneous CO_2 injections were used for conditions associated with peripheral arterial occlusion.

The rationale for using CO_2 against fat deposits grew out of earlier observations: lipid metabolism normalized in patients with atherosclerosis, and breakdown of fats and fat-like substances intensified under dry CO_2 baths. In 2004, a group of clinicians introduced injectable carboxytherapy as an adjunct after liposuction. The reason was practical: because adipose tissue can be unevenly distributed after surgery, small residual fat pads often remain, and these became a primary target for injected CO_2. At the same time, another clinically meaningful effect was noticed — skin treated with CO_2 tended to recover faster and more effectively.

CO_2 injections were found to support microcirculation, improving blood flow and, consequently, tissue oxygenation. They may also help downshift inflammation. Mechanistically, this is not surprising: our cells consume oxygen and release carbon dioxide, which acidifies the extracellular space. That shift signals red blood cells to offload oxygen more readily in the treated area, supporting increased perfusion and improved delivery of oxygen and nutrients.

On average, a course of carboxytherapy includes 15–20 sessions, with each session lasting about 15 min. The method is generally described as well-tolerated and safe.

In South America, Japan, and Europe, carboxytherapy is used not only for cellulite and post-liposuction recovery, but also to improve skin affected by stretch marks and hypertrophic scars, and to address periorbital dark circles. In the U.S., the overall stance is more cautious, and the FDA has not officially approved this technique.

More recently, a non-invasive form of carboxytherapy has appeared that uses a hydrogel matrix applied to the skin. The reagents react and release carbon dioxide. The gel then "traps" the CO_2, limiting its escape into the atmosphere. Over time, CO_2 concentration near the skin surface exceeds that on the other side of the barrier, and the gas diffuses passively into the epidermis and then into deeper layers.

A significant advantage of topical carboxytherapy is the absence of trauma and pain. However, when the goal is to influence deeper targets (fat deposits and vessels), topical delivery is typically less effective than injections. That is why injectable carboxytherapy is generally preferred for cellulite. For more superficial aesthetic and dermatologic goals — skin rejuvenation, acne and post-acne, rosacea, and scars — both injectable and non-invasive CO_2 delivery can be used effectively.

Carboxytherapy can be applied across different stages of cellulite via injections into affected areas. The total gas volume per session should be at least 160 cm^3 (about 20 cm^3 per injection), and it varies depending on the patient's skin status and the indication. In many cases, around 10 treatments are needed to see the desired change.

Patients should be counseled in advance that CO_2 introduction can cause moderate, short-lived localized discomfort because CO_2 bubbles can irritate pain receptors. Transient chills, itching or burning, and a sensation of fullness or heaviness are also possible.

Hyperemia may appear at the puncture site and can clearly outline the extent of CO_2 dispersion from the injection point. Gas emphysema can slightly lift the skin, creating a puffy look and a crackling (crepitant) sensation on palpation. These effects are temporary and typically subside within 15–30 min. To reduce these sensations in the injection zone, an anesthetic cream and vibration can be used (Sadala A.Y. et al., 2022).

Dermatologic effects of carboxytherapy (Oliveira S.M.D. et al., 2020; Bagherani N. et al., 2023; Susini P. et al., 2025):

- Reduction of fat deposits
- Improvement of skin elasticity and turgor
- Smoothing of skin topography
- Reduction of puffiness
- Evening of skin tone

Absolute contraindications to carboxytherapy:

- Epilepsy, hysteria, seizure disorders, pain syndromes, radicular syndromes, peripheral nerve injury (reduced skin sensitivity), and fear of injections

- Recent stroke or myocardial infarction
- Acute intoxication with alcohol or narcotic substances
- Cardiovascular disease, including paroxysmal tachycardia, atrial fibrillation, unstable angina, hypertension, vascular aneurysms, acute thrombophlebitis, embolism, and varicose veins
- Acute and chronic inflammatory skin conditions, including swelling, herpetic eruptions, local infections, dermatitis, and gangrene
- Tuberculosis
- Chronic diseases in an exacerbation or decompensation phase, as well as febrile conditions
- Endocrine disorders and marked abdominal obesity
- Pregnancy and breastfeeding
- Blood coagulation disorders and hematologic disease
- Tumors of any etiology

Part VI

Anti-cellulite cosmetic products

Cosmetic anti-cellulite products are widely available today, but their real-world effectiveness is often limited. The main reason is simple anatomy: topical ingredients cannot reliably reach adipocytes because these cells sit too deep. To get there, an ingredient would have to cross not only the *stratum corneum*, but also the epidermis and dermis. There are also regulatory boundaries that restrict cosmetics to effects within the skin's more superficial layers.

Still, cosmetics can be an excellent complement to intensive interventions targeting SAT and can play a meaningful role in a comprehensive anti-cellulite plan. They are used in professional treatments and are commonly recommended for supportive home care.

To improve the odds of penetration, several approaches are used:

- Adding transdermal carriers and penetration enhancers that temporarily increase *stratum corneum* permeability and help active ingredients pass through the skin's main barrier (Kassem A.A. et al., 2023).
- Wrapping: applying a product under an occlusive film. Occlusion reduces water evaporation, increases hydration within the *stratum corneum*, disrupts organization of the lipid barrier, and can increase permeability to active ingredients.
- Applying anti-cellulite products after chemical peels or mechanical exfoliation, which alters the *stratum corneum* structure.
- Applying specialized products after microneedling, which creates microchannels in the *stratum corneum* (Hameed H.I., Al-Mayahy M.H., 2024).
- Using energy-based delivery techniques such as electrophoresis and sonophoresis (Albash R. et al., 2024).

1.1. Active ingredients

What makes anti-cellulite formulations "anti-cellulite" is the targeted actives they contain. Below are some of the most common groups.

1.1.1. Stimulation of lipolysis

Because fat is a primary contributor to cellulite, agents that promote triglyceride breakdown inside adipocytes are considered core components of most anti-cellulite formulations. Common examples include (see Part V, section 1.2.1):

- **β-Adrenoreceptor stimulation**: plant alkaloids such as caffeine, theophylline, theobromine, and aminophylline (Fouad S.A. et al., 2024)
- **α2-Adrenoreceptor inhibition**: yohimbine
- **Phosphodiesterase inhibition**: caffeine, theophylline, and theobromine

These ingredients are often combined within a single formulation.

1.1.2. Fat burning

Stimulating lipolysis alone is usually not enough for durable results. If nothing else changes, free fatty acids will circulate and may eventually be stored again in the same depot. And if fatty acid transport into the bloodstream is limited, accumulation within adipocytes can further suppress lipolysis.

Many anti-cellulite products include ingredients positioned as mitochondrial "fat-burning" support — for example, L-carnitine and coenzyme A (CoA). However, their clinical impact in topical formulations remains unclear. In practice, cellulite management benefits from pairing skin-focused care with more reliable drivers of energy expenditure and circulation — namely, exercise.

1.1.3. Strengthening the collagen–elastin framework and improving the dermal structure

Connective-tissue degradation and fluid stagnation are essential contributors to cellulite. To counter these processes, silicon derivatives — specifically silanols (silicone-related molecules containing an alcoholic –OH group) — are used. Silanols may bind to collagen fibers, helping protect them from free radical damage and glycation. They are also described as supporting connective-tissue drainage, reducing inflammation, and promoting lipolysis.

To support dermal matrix renewal, remodeling peptides are used to trigger physiologic turnover, mirroring the body's natural regulation of breakdown and synthesis.

1.1.4 Reduction of edema, improvement of microcirculation

Vitamins K and P (rutin) and specific synthetic peptides are used for anti-edema effects. A well-known example is Eyeseryl® (INCI: Acetyl Tetrapeptide-5), which is described as strengthening vascular walls by influencing the formation of their connective tissue component. Although it was initially developed for periorbital edema, its use in anti-cellulite formulations is also considered reasonable.

1.1.5. Anti-cellulite complexes

In addition to single ingredients, anti-cellulite products often include biologically active complexes (Al Bader T. et al., 2012). A frequent example is **brown seaweed** — kelp and fucus. In English, these are typically grouped as "seaweeds." Commonly used species include *Laminaria japonica*, *L. ochroleuca*, *L. digitata*, *L. saccharina*, and *Fucus vesiculosis*.

Polysaccharides, vitamins, and trace elements (selenium, bromine, iron, manganese, etc.) found in brown seaweeds are described as:

- Stimulating β-adrenoreceptors and increasing lipolysis
- Supporting water–salt balance and interstitial fluid drainage
- Helping remove metabolic byproducts
- Improving skin and vascular tone

Another common group is **xanthine derivatives** (especially caffeine), used either in pure form or via botanical extracts, such as:

- Coffee (*Coffea arabica*): caffeine, theobromine
- Cocoa (*Theobroma cacao*): caffeine, theobromine
- Guarana (*Paullinia cupana*): caffeine, theophylline, xanthine, guanine, hypoxanthine
- Cola (*Cola acuminata*): caffeine, theobromine, colanine
- Tea (*Thea sinensis*): caffeine, theobromine, theophylline, xanthine, dimethylxanthine
- Yerba mate (*Ilex paraguariensis*): caffeine, theobromine

To support microcirculation, formulations often include plant extracts also used in anti-varicose care, such as horse chestnut (*Aesculus hippocastanum*), ginkgo (*Ginkgo biloba*), ivy (*Hedera helix*), centella (*Centella asiatica*), mountain arnica (*Arnica montana*), and needle thorn (*Ruscus aculeatus*).

Anti-cellulite creams also frequently contain **vegetable oils** (jojoba, wheat germ, evening primrose) and essential oils (lemon, bitter orange, oregano, lavender, myrtle, marjoram, coriander, chamomile, sage, bergamot, coniferous trees, sandalwood). Together, these components are used to stimulate peripheral lymphatic and blood flow, strengthen vessel walls, improve water and electrolite exchange and cellular metabolism, and soften the skin.

To support overall skin quality, formulations may include **antioxidant vitamins** C and E, along with **metabolism-supporting vitamins** B_5 and B_6, which are involved in epidermal renewal. Wheat germ or spirulina extracts are sometimes added as nutrient-rich bases.

1.2. Professional cosmetic treatments

1.2.1. Thalassotherapy

Thalassotherapy uses factors of the marine environment — climate, seawater, mud, algae, sand, and other sea-derived components — for therapeutic purposes (Antonelli M., Donelli D., 2025).

A course of thalassotherapy may support neuro- and endocrine regulation, which is essential for balancing lipolysis and lipogenesis and for regulating water–salt metabolism. When combined with diet, massage, aquatic procedures, exercise, and a positive emotional context, sea-based programs can reduce visible cellulite and ease tissue stagnation (Amuso D. et al., 2024). Marine resources rich in iodine are also considered beneficial for skin and overall health.

A 2-week thalassotherapy program at specialized resorts may offer lasting year-round benefits. However, resort-based care is not always accessible, so thalassotherapy has been adapted for local settings. While the warm sea climate cannot be "packaged", sea salts, muds, and algae can be concentrated, processed, and transported. Massage and hydrotherapy can be delivered essentially anywhere.

1.2.2. Mud therapy

Therapeutic mud is a complex natural biochemical material with multidirectional effects on the human body. Its composition varies by origin — it may be silt, sapropel, peat-based, and sourced from estuaries as well as salt and freshwater lakes.

Mud retains heat for extended periods and releases it gradually during treatment. With thermal exposure, vessels dilate, supporting blood and lymph flow. Therapeutic mud also contains biologically active components, including mineral and organic compounds, vitamins, and biogenic stimulants. Some elements can absorb skin secretions, contributing to cleansing (Hamed S., Almalty A.M., 2018).

1.2.3. Wraps

Wraps are a common adaptation of thalassotherapy and mud therapy. In modern aesthetic practice, wraps made from brown seaweed — often combined with other botanicals — are widely used, typically together with massage and with scrubs, peels, lotions, sprays, or creams applied before and/or after the wrap.

Peels and scrubs prepare the skin by cleansing pores and removing corneocytes, thereby enhancing the wrap's effect. After cleansing, the treatment product (cream- or mud-based) is applied to the target zones, and the body is wrapped in a dedicated film. Wrap duration varies, but averages about 45 min. Temperature is a key active factor, and wraps are commonly grouped as:

- Isothermal (maintaining body temperature)
- Hot (thermoactive)
- Cold

Hot wraps create a sauna-like effect that can increase penetration of active substances into the skin. Formulations for hot wraps vary, but often include salt concentrates or sea clay, plus extracts of brown algae, ivy, horse chestnut, and other botanicals, along with essential oils. With rising temperature, these substances can markedly increase blood flow and exert complex vasoactive effects. However, thermoactive wraps are not suitable for everyone and are generally not recommended for patients with varicose veins, couperose, or other vascular conditions.

Cold wraps are commonly used when vascular status is compromised.

To enhance outcomes and improve delivery toward the hypodermis, wraps are often combined with manual anti-cellulite massage. This supports blood flow and lymphatic drainage in vessels surrounding adipose tissue. Massage should be prescribed and performed by trained specialists, with contraindications carefully considered.

Part VII

Other methods for body contouring

1.1. Nutraceuticals

Nutritional correction, including the use of selected nutraceuticals, is an essential part of addressing excess weight and maintaining a healthy weight. At the same time, cellulite and localized fat deposits can appear even in people with a slender build. For that reason, supplements that influence lipid metabolism and support the reduction of lipid deposits are more accurately described as weight loss aids rather than "anti-cellulite supplements".

Despite growing interest in nutritional supplements, responsible skincare professionals should remember that selecting nutraceuticals and designing a plan for weight loss and weight maintenance falls within the expertise of a nutritionist (Sergeev I.N. et al., 2020). While this is a valuable element of a body contouring program, it should be planned by a nutritionist rather than an aesthetic practitioner (Watanabe M. et al., 2020; Batsis J.A. et al., 2021; Dini I., Mancusi A., 2023).

Many ingredients used in topical products also appear in weight management supplements. Examples include extracts of kelp and fucus, as well as sources of bioflavonoids such as ginkgo leaf extract, various parts of Centella asiatica (often called gotu kola), grape seed, and maritime pine bark. These ingredients are positioned to strengthen the walls of blood and lymphatic vessels while supporting peripheral circulation. Some anti-cellulite formulas also include hawthorn extract to support central circulation.

A common component of anti-cellulite capsules is evening primrose (*Oenothera biennis*) oil, which supports overall skin health. Rosemary (*Rosmarinus officinalis*) extract or oil may increase cutaneous blood flow and is also reported to support liver function and the body's detoxification pathways. Turmeric (*Curcuma longa*) extract is used to support digestion, while dandelion extract is positioned to support digestion and urinary function. Mate tea extract (from *Ilex paraguariensis*) is described as supporting digestion, urination, metabolism, and muscle tone. Extracts of horse chestnut (*Aesculus hippocastanum*), mountain arnica (*Arnica montana*), and butcher's broom (*Ruscus aculeatus*) are also used to support peripheral circulation, improve tone, and may increase adipocyte membrane permeability.

Vitamins often found in anti-cellulite formulas are antioxidant vitamins C and E, as well as vitamins B_5 and B_6, which are crucial for regular skin cell renewal.

Relying solely on nutraceuticals for weight loss, without additional body-contouring methods, is ineffective. However, they can complement a comprehensive physiologic program and work alongside other techniques.

1.2. Drugs for blood sugar control and weight loss

In recent years, semaglutide, tirzepatide, liraglutide, and their analogs have attracted substantial attention in the media, on blogs, and on forums. These synthetic medications are primarily intended for people with type 2 diabetes mellitus, used alongside diet and exercise to improve glycemic control (Shareef L.G. et al., 2024). Administered subcutaneously, they can support both blood glucose regulation and weight loss, leading to their use as weight-loss aids among some non-diabetic individuals (Carboni A. et al., 2024).

This pathway accelerated in 2012, when Novo Nordisk, a Danish pharmaceutical company, launched semaglutide, a synthetic glucagon-like peptide 1 (GLP-1) agonist. Semaglutide is 94% similar to endogenous GLP-1 and binds to GLP-1 receptors, thereby mimicking its effects. This receptor interaction is associated with several clinically relevant actions:

- **Glucose-lowering:** Semaglutide stimulates insulin secretion and suppresses glucagon production (a hormone that raises blood glucose) only when glucose levels are elevated.

- **Appetite control:** It influences central hunger and satiety pathways, reducing perceived hunger.
- **Delayed gastric emptying:** This increases post-meal fullness and can further support weight loss.

Overall, these medications can improve glycemic control in patients with type 2 diabetes and support weight loss in some individuals. Unlike endogenous GLP-1, semaglutide is more resistant to degradation by dipeptidyl peptidase-4 (DPP-4), which helps prolong its activity in the body.

The first widely available semaglutide-based medication is Ozempic. Ozempic is supplied as an injectable solution for subcutaneous administration. The recommended starting dose is 0.25 mg once a week, which may be increased to 0.5 mg or 1.0 mg once a week as needed, under physician supervision. The maximum allowed dose is 1.0 mg. Injections may be given in the abdomen, thigh, or upper arm, ideally at the same time each week, as directed by the physician. Maintaining a gular schedule and avoiding missed doses is essential.

Clinical studies report that Ozempic supports:

- Significant reductions in blood glucose and glycated hemoglobin HbA1c
- Weight loss, which is particularly relevant for patients who are overweight
- Improved pancreatic beta cell function
- Reduced risk of cardiovascular complications in the presence of pertinent risk factors

The most frequently reported **short-term adverse effects** include:

- Nausea, vomiting
- Diarrhea
- Abdominal pain
- Headache
- Injection site reactions: itching, redness, or swelling

Another commonly discussed effect is facial aging, also known as the "Ozempic face." It is described as sharper facial contours, more visible wrinkles, and lax, sagging skin. These changes are attributed to rapid weight loss, reduced SAT volume, and excess stretched skin. This effect is not unique to Ozempic and can be seen after any fast weight loss, regardless of cause.

In rare cases, serious **longer-term complications** such as pancreatitis, cholecystitis, gastroparesis, intestinal obstruction, and anterior ischemic optic neuropathy may occur. While only isolated cases have been reported in the literature, these events represent a clinically significant risk (Tan H.C. et al., 2022). Therefore, Ozempic and its analogs should be used only under physician supervision.

1.3. Specialized clothing

Specialized garments — belts, bodysuits, corsets, and leggings — are sometimes used to support aesthetic programs aimed at reducing the appearance of cellulite. Compression garments are popular, but it is essential to remember that excessive or prolonged compression can impair microcirculation and contribute to increased adipocyte hypertrophy.

As functional textiles have advanced — fabrics designed to influence skin condition — a new category of anti-cellulite clothing has appeared. These garments are produced using fabrics impregnated with active substances with anti-cellulite effects, such as caffeine (Zornoza B. et al., 2022; Pina-Vidal C. et al., 2024). Products made from multilayer textiles that create a sauna-like effect are also available.

Conclusion

Effective SAT remodeling is no longer theoretical — it is now a practical reality, driven by significant advances in adipose-tissue biology and physiology over the last 20 years. Findings that were previously hard to explain now make sense, and we have a much clearer view of the fine regulatory mechanisms that shape adipocyte function. That progress has accelerated the development of both surgical options and non-surgical aesthetic interventions targeting adipose tissue. In parallel, investigators have developed research tools that support meaningful quantitative and qualitative comparisons across different intervention types. This kind of evidence is essential when you are building comprehensive programs that truly fit the individual.

Lipomodeling is increasingly becoming a distinct field with all the hallmarks of a mature discipline: a scientific foundation, a growing evidence base, expanding diagnostic and research capabilities, and a widening set of therapeutic technologies. Within this framework, clinicians can address a broad spectrum of aesthetic concerns and relevant pathologic conditions.

When discussing cellulite, it is essential to remember that it is often more a common feature of the female body — and a variant of normal — than a severe disease (we are not referring to extreme clinical stages). It is also commonly approached as an aesthetic concern. Accordingly, an effective anti-cellulite strategy is best built around physiologic restoration: supporting lipolysis, limiting lipogenesis, improving blood and lymph flow, reducing congestion, increasing vascular tone, and strengthening vessel walls. Consistent skin care in affected zones also matters. Improving tissue structure, maintaining muscle, and supporting metabolic activity can reduce volume and noticeably enhance the appearance of cellulite-prone skin. At the same time, these efforts may fall short if dietary patterns do not change and a sedentary lifestyle persists.

References

Abraira V.E., Ginty D.D. The sensory neurons of touch. Neuron 2013; 79(4): 618–639.

Adams J.E., Foster J.H., Faulk W.H. et al. Experimental production of subcutaneous fat necrosis by general hypothermia; relation to the chemical composition of fat. Surg Forum 1955; 5: 556–563.

Al-Mutairi N., Nour T. The effect of weight reduction on treatment outcomes in obese patients with psoriasis on biologic therapy: a randomized controlled prospective trial. Expert Opin Biol Ther 2014; 14(6): 749–756.

Albash R., Abdelbari M.A., Elbesh R.M. et al. Sonophoresis mediated diffusion of caffeine loaded Transcutol® enriched cerosomes for topical management of cellulite. Eur J Pharm Sci 2024; 201: 106875.

Ali Y.H. Laser-assisted lipolysis burn safety: proposed detailed parameters with assessment of their efficacy and safety. Plast Reconstr Surg Glob Open 2018; 6(10): e1934.

Alizadeh Z., Halabchi F., Mazaheri R. et al. Review of the mechanisms and effects of noninvasive body contouring devices on cellulite and subcutaneous fat. Int J Endocrinol Metab 2016; 14(4): e36727.

Allam N.M., Elshorbagy R.T., Eid M.M. et al. Comparison of extracorporeal shock wave therapy versus manual lymphatic drainage on cellulite after liposuction: a randomized clinical trial. Evid Based Complement Alternat Med 2021; 2021: 9956879.

Amuso D., Medoro A., Scapagnini G. et al. A pilot study on the efficacy of a seaweed mud application in the treatment of cellulite. J Cosmet Dermatol 2024; 23(6): 2181–2189.

Antonelli M., Donelli D. A narrative review of thalassotherapy and the health benefits of seawater and coastal climates. Int J Biometeorol 2025; 69(3): 517–526.

Armstrong A.W., Harskamp C.T., Armstrong E.J. The association between psoriasis and obesity: a systematic review and meta-analysis of observational studies. Nutr Diabetes 2012; 2(12): e54.

Arshakyan V.A. Commentary on the article "Who is last? Different approaches to radiofrequency-associated liposuction." Apparatnaya Kosmetologiya 2020; 3: 68–81.

Atieh B., Baajour J., El Merkabaoui H., Makkawi K. Literature review and evidence-based comparative analysis of traditional suction-assisted lipectomy (SAL) vs. ultrasound-assisted liposuction (UAL) reported outcomes. Aesthetic Plast Surg 2025; 49(16): 4648–4655.

Bachelor E., Moradi A., Stevens G. et al. Safety, effectiveness, and participant satisfaction with multiple simultaneous cryolipolysis treatments using a dual-applicator cryolipolysis system. Dermatol Surg 2025; 51(6): 604–610.

Bagherani N., Smoller B.R., Tavoosidana G. et al. An overview of the role of carboxytherapy in dermatology. J Cosmet Dermatol 2023; 22(9): 2399-2407.

Bass L.S., Kaminer M.S. Insights into the pathophysiology of cellulite: a review. Dermatol Surg 2020; 46 Suppl 1(1): S77–S85.

Batsis J.A., Apolzan J.W., Bagley P.J. et al. A systematic review of dietary supplements and alternative therapies for weight loss. Obesity (Silver Spring) 2021; 29(7): 1102–1113.

Beidas O.E., Gusenoff J.A. Update on liposuction: what all plastic surgeons should know. Plast Reconstr Surg 2021; 147(4): 658e–668e.

Bellini E., Grieco M.P., Raposio E. A journey though liposuction and liposculture: Review. Ann Med Surg. 2017; 6(24): 53–60.

Belzer F.O., Southard J.H. Principles of solid-organ preservation by cold storage. Transplant 1988; 45(4): 673–676.

Bergsbaken T., Fink S.L., Cookson B.T. Pyroptosis: host cell death and inflammation. Nat Rev Microbiol 2009; 7(2): 99–109.

Boey G.E., Wasilenchuk J.L. Enhanced clinical outcome with manual massage following cryolipolysis treatment: A 4-month study of safety and efficacy. Lasers Surg Med 2014; 46: 20–26.

Bora P., Majumdar A.S. Adipose tissue-derived stromal vascular fraction in regenerative medicine: a brief review on biology and translation. Stem Cell Res Ther 2017; 8(1): 145.

Cannon J., Rajakaruna G., Dyer J. et al. Severe lower limb cellulitis: defining the epidemiology and risk factors for primary episodes in a population-based case-control study. Clin Microbiol Infect 2018; 24(10): 1089–1094.

Cao L., Gou X., Song L. et al. Spatial evolution mechanism of coal structure damage and gas permeability under waterbased ultrasonic treatment. Environ Earth Sci 2024; 83: 299.

Carboni A., Woessner S., Martini O. et al. Natural weight loss or "Ozempic Face": demystifying a social media phenomenon. J Drugs Dermatol 2024; 23(1): 1367–1368.

Carobbio S., Guénantin A.C., Samuelson I. et al. Brown and beige fat: from molecules to physiology and pathophysiology. Biochim Biophys Acta Mol Cell Biol Lipids 2019; 1864(1): 37–50.

Caruso M.K., Roberts A.T., Bissoon L. et al. An evaluation of mesotherapy solutions for inducing lipolysis and treating cellulite. J Plast Reconstr Aesthet Surg 2008; 61(11): 1321–1324.

Casabona G., Pereira G. Microfocused ultrasound with visualization and calcium hydroxylapatite for improving skin laxity and cellulite appearance. Plast Reconstr Surg Glob Open 2017; 25;5(7): e1388.

Catalán V., Gómez-Ambrosi J., Ramírez B. et al. Increased expression levels of PIEZO1 in visceral adipose tissue in obesity and type 2 diabetes are triggered by mechanical forces and are associated with inflammation. Mol Med 2024; 30(1): 255.

Celik N., Turgut E., Yilmaz B. Design analysis of an implant and antenna system by using Taguchi method. Heat Mass Transfer 2018; 54: 10.1007/s00231-017-2143-z.

Chang S.J., Hsu S.C., Tien K.J. et al. Metabolic syndrome associated with toenail onychomycosis in Taiwanese with diabetes mellitus. Int J Dermatol 2008; 47(5): 467–472.

Chen P.Y., Cripps A.W., West N.P. et al. A correlation-based network for biomarker discovery in obesity with metabolic syndrome. BMC Bioinformatics 2019; 20(Suppl 6): 477.

Cheng N., Van Hoof H., Bockx E. et al. The effects of electric currents on ATP generation, protein synthesis, and membrane transport of rat skin. Clin Orthop Relat Res 1982; (171): 264–272.

Conte M., Martucci M., Sandri M. et al. The dual role of the pervasive "fattish" tissue remodeling with age. Front Endocrinol (Lausanne) 2019; 10: 114.

Cousin B., Casteilla L., Lafontan M. et al. Local sympathetic denervation of white adipose tissue in rats induces preadipocyte proliferation without noticeable changes in metabolism. Endocrinol 1993; 133(5): 2255–2262.

de Farias Pires T., Azambuja A.P., Horimoto A.R. et al. A population-based study of the stratum corneum moisture. Clin Cosmet Investig Dermatol 2016; 9: 79–87.

Decorato J., Chen B., Sierra R. Subcutaneous adipose tissue response to a non-invasive hyperthermic treatment using a 1,060 nm laser. Lasers Surg Med 2017; 49(5): 480–489.

Dini I., Mancusi A. Weight loss supplements. Molecules 2023; 28(14): 5357.

Downie J., Kaspar M. Contactless abdominal fat reduction with Selective RF™ evaluated by magnetic resonance imaging (MRI): case study. J Drugs Dermatol 2016; 15(4): 491–495.

Duncan D., Rubin J.P., Golitz L. et al. Refinement of technique in injection lipolysis based on scientific studies and clinical evaluation. Clin Plast Surg 2009; 36(2):195–209, v-vi; discussion 211–213.

Duncan D.I. (ed.) Enhanced Liposuction: New Perspectives and Techniques. Intechopen, 2022.

Duncan D.I. Combination treatment for buttock and abdominal remodeling and skin improvement using HIFEM procedure and simultaneous delivery of radiofrequency and targeted pressure energy. J Cosmet Dermatol 2021; 20(12): 3893–3898.

Duncan D.I., Hasengschwandtner F. Lipodissolve for subcutaneous fat reduction and skin retraction. Aesthet Surg J 2005; 25(5): 530–543.

Dupont E., Journet M., Oula M.L. et al. An integral topical gel for cellulite reduction: results from a double-blind, randomized, placebo-controlled evaluation of efficacy. Clin Cosmet Investig Dermatol 2014; 7: 73–88.

Elhelf I.A.S., Albahar H., Shah U. et al. High-intensity focused ultrasound: the fundamentals, clinical applications, and research trends. Diagn Interv Imaging 2018; 99(6): 349–359.

Emanuele E., Minoretti P., Altabas K. et al. Adiponectin expression in subcutaneous adipose tissue is reduced in women with cellulite. Int J Dermatol 2011; 50(4): 412–416.

Epstein E.H., Oren M.E. Popsicle panniculitis. N Engl J Med 1970; 82: 966–967.

Esteve Ràfols M. Adipose tissue: cell heterogeneity and functional diversity. Endocrinol Nutr 2014; 61(2): 100–112.

Fagien S., McChesney P., Subramanian M., Jones D.H. Prevention and management of injection-related adverse effects in facial aesthetics: considerations for ATX-101 (Deoxycholic Acid Injection) treatment. Dermatol Surg 2016; 42(Suppl 1): S300–S304.

Fajkošová K., Machovcová A., Onder M., Fritz K. Selective radiofrequency therapy as a non-invasive approach for contactless body contouring and circumferential reduction. J Drugs Dermatol 2014; 13(3): 291–296.

Fakiha K. Adipose stromal vascular fraction: a promising treatment for severe burn injury. Hum Cell 2022; 35(5): 1323–1337.

Ferraro G.A., De Francesco F., Cataldo C. et al. Synergistic effects of cryolipolysis and shock waves for noninvasive body contouring. Aesthetic Plast Surg 2012; 36(3): 667–679.

Ferreli C., Pinna A.L., Pilloni L. et al. Obesity-associated lymphedematous mucinosis: two further cases and review of the literature. Dermatopathology (Basel) 2018; 5(1): 16–20.

Few J., Saltz R., Beaty M. et al. Cryolipolysis: clinical best practices and other nonclinical considerations. Aesthet Surg J Open Forum 2020; 2(2): ojaa010.

Fong G.H. Regulation of angiogenesis by oxygen sensing mechanisms. J Mol Med (Berl). 2009; 87(6): 549–60.

Fouad S.A., Badr T.A., Abdelbary A. et al. New insight for enhanced topical targeting of caffeine for effective cellulite treatment: in vitro characterization, permeation studies, and histological evaluation in rats. AAPS PharmSciTech 2024; 25(7): 237.

Franco W., Kothare A., Ronan S.J. et al. Hyperthermic injury to adipocyte cells by selective heating of subcutaneous fat with a novel radiofrequency device: feasibility studies. Lasers Surg Med 2010; 42(5): 361–370.

Friedmann D.P., Kommera J., Durga P. et al. Evaluating real-world use and adverse events from 3262 patients treated with 18,203 cycles of cryolipolysis for localized fat reduction: a multilocation practice retrospective chart review. Aesthet Surg J 2025; 45(5): 493–500.

Friedmann D.P., Vick G.L., Mishra V. Cellulite: a review with a focus on subcision. Clin Cosmet Investig Dermatol 2017; 10: 17–23.

Frigolet M.E., Gutiérrez-Aguilar R. The colors of adipose tissue. Gac Med Mex 2020; 156(2): 142–149.

Fritz K., Salavastru C. Long-term follow-up on patients treated for abdominal fat using a selective contactless radiofrequency device. J Cosmet Dermatol. 2017; 16(4): 471–475.

Gabriel A., Chan V., Caldarella M. et al. Cellulite: current understanding and treatment. Aesthet Surg J Open Forum. 2023; 5: ojad050.

Gaidash N.V. A comprehensive approach to body contour correction: the Body to Life program with BTL devices. Apparatnaya Kosmetologiya 2020; 1: 9–23.

Gao Y., Qimuge N.R., Qin J. et al. Acute and chronic cold exposure differentially affects the browning of porcine white adipose tissue. Animal 2018; 12(7): 1435–1441.

Garibyan L., Cornelissen L., Sipprell W. et al. Transient alterations of cutaneous sensory nerve function by noninvasive cryolipolysis. J Invest Dermatol 2015; 135(11): 2623–2631.

Garibyan L., Moradi Tuchayi S., Javorsky E. et al. Subcutaneous fat reduction with injected ice slurry. Plast Reconstr Surg 2020; 145(4): 725e–733e.

Geeta Sai G., Thillaikkarasi A., Wahab A.J. Obesity-related skin conditions: exploring the link. Cureus 2024; 16(4): e57772.

Goldberg D.J. Adipocyte apoptosis following a novel method for double chin reduction: a pilot human histology study. J Cosmet Dermatol 2025; 24(1): e16643.

Greenwald E., Christman M., Penn L. et al. Cold panniculitis: Adverse cutaneous effect of whole-body cryotherapy. JAAD Case Rep 2018; 4(4): 344–345.

Gudipaty S.A., Lindblom J., Loftus P.D. et al. Mechanical stretch triggers rapid epithelial cell division through Piezo1. Nature 2017; 543(7643): 118–121.

Guida B., Nino M., Perrino N.R. et al. The impact of obesity on skin disease and epidermal permeability barrier status. J Eur Acad Dermatol Venereol 2010; 24(2): 191–195.

Guida S., Zerbinati N., Conforti C. et al. From cellulite to post-liposuction skin irregularities: a proposal for definition and classification. J Clin Aesthet Dermatol 2025; 18(3): 39–41.

Guillaume-Jugnot P., Daumas A., Magalon J. et al. Autologous adipose-derived stromal vascular fraction in patients with systemic sclerosis: 12-month follow-up. Rheumatology (Oxford) 2016; 55(2): 301–306.

Halaas Y., Bernardy J. Mechanism of nonthermal induction of apoptosis by high-intensity focused electromagnetic procedure: Biochemical investigation in a porcine model. J Cosmet Dermatol 2020; 19(3): 605–611.

Hamed S., Almalty A.M. Skin tolerance of three types of Dead Sea mud on healthy skin: a short-term study. J Cosmet Sci 2018; 69(4): 269–278.

Hameed H.I., Al-Mayahy M.H. Combined approach of nanoemulgel and microneedle pretreatment as a topical anticellulite therapy. ADMET DMPK 2024; 12(6): 903–923.

Han X., Yang M., Yin B. et al. The efficacy and safety of subcutaneous radiofrequency after liposuction: a new application for face and neck skin tightening. Aesthet Surg J 2021; 41(3): NP94–NP100.

Hansson E., Svensson H., Brorson H. Review of Dercum's disease and proposal of diagnostic criteria, diagnostic methods, classification and management. Orphanet J Rare Dis 2012; 7: 23.

Hausman D.B., DiGirolamo M., Bartness T.J. et al. The biology of white adipocyte proliferation. Obes Rev 2001; 2(4): 239–254.

Haxthausen H. Adiponecrosis e frigore. Br J Dermatol. 1941; 53: 83–89.

He L., Si G., Huang J. et al. Mechanical regulation of stem-cell differentiation by the stretchactivated Piezo channel. Nature 2018; 555(7694): 103–106.

He N., Liu M., Wu Y. Adipose tissue and hematopoiesis: Friend or foe? J Clin Lab Anal 2023; 37(6): e24872.

Hedayati B., Juhász M., Chu S., Mesinkovska N.A. Adverse events associated with cryolipolysis: a systematic review of the literature. Dermatol Surg 2020; 46(Suppl 1): S8–S13.

Hirt P.A., Castillo DE., Yosipovitch G., Keri J.E. Skin changes in the obese patient. J Am Acad Dermatol 2019; 81(5): 1037–1057.

Hochsinger C. Über eine akute kongelative zellgewebsverhärtung in der submentalregion bei kindern. Mschr Kinderheilk 1902; 1: 323–327.

Hoefflin S.M. Hypotonic Pharmacological Lipo-Dissolution. Perspect Plast Surg 1999; 13: 85–98.

Hoefflin S.M. Lipoplasty with hypotonic pharmacologic lipo-dissolution. Aesthet Surg J 2002; 22(6): 1321–1324.

Hoffmann C., Weigert C. Skeletal muscle as an endocrine organ: the role of myokines in exercise adaptations. Cold Spring Harb Perspect Med 2017; 7(11): a029793.

Huang Z., Huang Y., Ning X. et al. The functional effects of Piezo channels in mesenchymal stem cells. Stem Cell Res Ther 2023; 14(1): 222.

Humphrey J.D., Dufresne E.R., Schwartz M.A. Mechanotransduction and extracellular matrix homeostasis. Nat Rev Mol Cell Biol 2014; 15(12): 802–812.

Huttunen R., Syrjanen J. Obesity and the risk and outcome of infection. Int J Obes (Lond) 2013; 37(3): 333–340.

Hwang I.C., Kim K.K., Lee K.R. Cryolipolysis-induced abdominal fat change: split-body trials. PLoS One 2020; 15(12): e0242782.

Ingargiola M.J., Motakef S., Chung M.T. et al. Cryolipolysis for fat reduction and body contouring: safety and efficacy of current treatment paradigms. Plast Reconstr Surg 2015; 135(6): 1581–1590.

Jackson R.F., Stern F.A., Neira R. et al. Application of low-level laser therapy for noninvasive body contouring. Lasers Surg Med 2012; 44(3): 211–217.

Jacob C., Weiss R.A. Simultaneous HIFEM and synchronized RF procedure can be effectively used for increasing muscle mass and decreasing fat in the upper arm. J Clin Aesthet Dermatol 2023; 16(2): 50–54.

Jacob C.I., Rank B. Abdominal remodeling in postpartum women by using a high-intensity focused electromagnetic (HIFEM) procedure: an investigational magnetic resonance imaging (MRI) pilot study. J Clin Aesthet Dermatol 2020; 13(9 Suppl 1): S16–S20.

Jafarzadeh A., Pour Mohammad A., Keramati H. et al. Regenerative medicine in the treatment of specific dermatologic disorders: a systematic review of randomized controlled clinical trials. Stem Cell Res Ther 2024; 15(1): 176.

Jalian H.R., Avram M.M. Cryolipolysis: a historical perspective and current clinical practice. Semin Cutan Med Surg 2013; 32(1): 31–34.

Jalian H.R., Avram M.M., Garibyan L. et al. Paradoxical adipose hyperplasia after cryolipolysis. JAMA Dermatol 2014; 150(3): 317–319.

Kandula P., Javorsky E., Austen W.G. Jr., Kaminer M.S. Injection cryolipolysis: first-in-human Study. Plast Reconstr Surg Glob Open 2021; 9(9): e3818.

Kassem A.A., Asfour M.H., Abd El-Alim S.H. et al. Topical caffeine-loaded nanostructured lipid carriers for enhanced treatment of cellulite: A 32 full factorial design optimization and in vivo evaluation in rats. Int J Pharm 2023; 643: 123271.

Kaur H., Reyes-Barron C., Sipprell W.H. et al. Painful purulent nodules caused by Mycobacterium at site of Lipodissolve injections. Am J Dermatopathol 2022; 44(4): 257–259.

Kefauver J.M., Ward A.B., Patapoutian A. Discoveries in structure and physiology of mechanically activated ion channels. Nature 2020; 587(7835): 567–576.

Kelly E., Rodriguez-Feliz J., Kelly M.E. Paradoxical adipose hyperplasia after cryolipolysis: a report on incidence and common factors identified in 510 patients. Plast Reconstr Surg 2016; 137(3): 639e–640e.

Kennedy J., Verne S., Griffith R. et al. Non-invasive subcutaneous fat reduction: a review. J Eur Acad Dermatol Venereol 2015; 29(9): 1679–1688.

Kershaw E.E., Flier J.S. Adipose tissue as an endocrine organ. J Clin Endocrinol Metab 2004; 89(6): 2548–2556.

Khalil S., Galadari H.I. Cellulite: an update on pathogenesis and management. Dermatol Clin 2024; 42(1): 129–137.

Kim D., Kwon S. Vibrational stress affects extracellular signal-regulated kinases activation and cytoskeleton structure in human keratinocytes. PLoS ONE 2020; 15(4): e0231174.

Kim M., Kim K.E., Jeong S.W. et al. Effects of the ultra-high-frequency electrical field radiofrequency device on mouse skin: a histologic and molecular study. Plast Reconstr Surg 2016; 138(2): 248e–255e.

Kim M., Lim J., Bae J.M., Park H.J. A pilot study of the efficacy of the POLARGEN ultra-highfrequency electric field (40.68 MHz) radiofrequency device in the treatment of facial contouring. J Cosmet Laser Ther 2017; 19(7): 404–408.

Klein K.B., Bachelor E.P., Becker E.V., Bowes L.E. Multiple same day cryolipolysis treatments for the reduction of subcutaneous fat are safe and do not affect serum lipid levels or liver function tests. Lasers Surg Med 2017; 49(7): 640–644.

Knobloch K., Kraemer R. Extracorporeal shock wave therapy (ESWT) for the treatment of cellulite—a current metaanalysis. Int J Surg 2015; 24(Pt B): 210–217.

Kosir J., Vella D., Jezersek M. Non-contact monitoring of the depth temperature profile for medical laser scanning technologies. Sci Rep 2020; 10(1): 20242.

Kostecka A., Kalamon N., Skoniecka A. et al. Adipose-derived mesenchymal stromal cells in clinical trials: Insights from single-cell studies. Life Sci 2024; 351: 122761.

Kwon T.R., Kim J.H., Jang Y.N. et al. Comparison of different energy response for lipolysis using a 1,060-nm laser: An animal study of three pigs. Skin Res Technol 2021; 27(1): 5–14.

Lafontan M. Adipose tissue and adipocyte dysregulation. Diabetes Metab 2014; 40(1): 16–28.

Lafontan M. Advances in adipose tissue metabolism. Int J Obes (Lond) 2008; 32(7): 39–51.

Lafontan M., Langin D. Lipolysis and lipid mobilization in human adipose tissue. Prog Lipid Res 2009; 48(5): 275–297.

Lee J.Y., Oh SW., Ryu H.Y., Seo Y.S. Development of a minimally invasive and non-invasive lipolysis laser system for effective fat reduction. J Lasers Med Sci 2021; 12: e55.

Lee Y.H., Mottillo E.P., Granneman J.G. Adipose tissue plasticity from WAT to BAT and in between. Biochim Biophys Acta 2014; 1842(3): 358–369.

Li J., Daly E., Campioli E. et al. De novo synthesis of steroids and oxysterols in adipocytes. J Biol Chem 2014; 289(2): 747–764.

Li P., Jin H., Liu D. et al. Study on the effect of leptin on fibroblast proliferation and collagen synthesis in vitro in rats. Zhongguo Xiu Fu Chong Jian Wai Ke Za Zhi 2005; 19(1): 20–22.

Li S., Cho E., Drucker A.M. et al. Obesity and risk for incident rosacea in US women. J Am Acad Dermatol 2017; 77(6): 1083–1087.

Lopes-Martins R.A.B., Barbosa L.V., Sousa M.M.B. et al. The effects of body cold exposure (cryolipolysis) on fat mass and plasma cholesterol. Life (Basel) 2024; 14(9): 1082.

Mahmud K., Crutchfield C.E. Lipodissolve for body sculpting: safety, effectiveness, and patient satisfaction. J Clin Aesthet Dermatol 2012; 5(10): 16–19.

Manstein D., Laubach H., Watanabe K. et al. Selective cryolysis: a novel method of noninvasive fat removal. Lasers Surg Med 2008; 40(9): 595–604.

Mantovani G.P., Marra C., De Maria F. et al. Adipose-derived stromal vascular fraction (SVF) for the treatment of androgenic alopecia (AGA): a systematic review. Acta Biomed 2023; 94(5): e2023236.

Manzano-Finol A., Parra-Pelosi H., Cubillos-Valencia G. et al. Laser-assisted lipolysis: a promising alternative to traditional liposuction. Aesthetic Plast Surg 2025 Aug 6. Epub ahead of print.

Marques M.A., Combes M., Roussel B. et al. Impact of a mechanical massage on gene expression profile and lipid mobilization in female gluteofemoral adipose tissue. Obes Facts 2011; 4(2): 121–129.

Mbiine R., Wayengera M., Ocan M. et al. Adipose-derived stromal vascular fraction (SVF) in scar treatment: a systematic review protocol. Am J Stem Cells 2022; 11(4): 56–63.

Menon A., Shauly O., Marxen T. et al. A clinical guide to the treatment of cellulite and comprehensive review of the etiology, pathophysiology, and utility of intervention. Aesthetic Plast Surg 2024; 48(10): 1985–1992.

Meyer P.F., da Silva RM., Oliveira G. et al. Effects of cryolipolysis on abdominal adiposity. Case Rep Dermatol Med 2016; 2016: 6052194.

Michon A. Shockwave therapy for the prevention of paradoxical adipose hyperplasia after cryolipolysis: myth or reality? Aesthet Surg J 2021; 41(8): NP1137–NP1138.

Mileva K., Georgieva B., Radicheva N. About the biological effects of high and extremely high frequency electromagnetic fields. Acta Physiol Pharmacol Bulg 2003; 27(2–3): 89–100.

Miron T.R., Flood E.D., Tykocki N.R. et al. Identification of Piezo1 channels in perivascular adipose tissue (PVAT) and their potential role in vascular function. Pharmacol Res 2022; 175: 105995.

Mo Y.Y., Han Y.X., Xu S. et al. Adipose tissue plasticity: a comprehensive definition and multidimensional insight. Biomolecules 2024; 14(10): 1223.

Modena D.A.O., Soares C.D., Martignago C.C.S. et al. Effects of LED photobiomodulation therapy on the subcutaneous fatty tissue of obese individuals — histological and immunohistochemical analysis. J Cosmet Laser Ther 2022; 24(6–8): 84–90.

Monteux C., Lafontan M. Use of the microdialysis technique to assess lipolytic responsiveness of femoral adipose tissue after 12 sessions of mechanical massage technique. J Eur Acad Dermatol Venereol 2008; 22(12): 1465–1470.

Moon K.C., Chung H.Y., Han S.K. et al. Possibility of injecting adipose-derived stromal vascular fraction cells to accelerate microcirculation in ischemic diabetic feet: a pilot study. Int J Stem Cells 2019; 12(1): 107–113.

Moonen M.P.B., Nascimento E.B.M., van Marken Lichtenbelt W.D. Human brown adipose tissue: underestimated target in metabolic disease? Biochim Biophys Acta Mol Cell Biol Lipids 2019; 1864(1): 104–112.

Neira R., Arroyave J., Ramirez H. et al. Fat liquefaction: effect of low-level laser energy on adipose tissue. Plast Reconstr Surg 2002; 110(3): 912–925.

Ni H., Liu C., Kong L. et al. Preparation of injectable porcine skin-derived collagen and its application in delaying skin aging by promoting the adhesion and chemotaxis of skin fibroblasts. Int J Biol Macromol 2023; 253(Pt 2): 126718.

Ni P., Farinelli W.A., Cheng L.L. et al. Total ice content and lipid saturation determine adipose tissue cryolipolysis by injection of ice-slurry. Lasers Surg Med 2023; 55(1): 116–125.

Nie T., Lu J., Zhang H., Mao L. Latest advances in the regulatory genes of adipocyte thermogenesis. Front Endocrinol (Lausanne) 2023; 14: 1250487.

Nikolis A., Enright K.M. A Multicenter evaluation of paradoxical adipose hyperplasia following cryolipolysis for fat reduction and body contouring: a review of 8658 cycles in 2114 patients. Aesthet Surg J 2021; 41(8): 932–941.

Nishioka M.A., Brassolatti P., Alves A.C.A. et al. Clinical protocol effects with led photobiomodulation for reducing adipose tissue in the abdomen region. J Cosmet Dermatol 2025; 24(2): e16675.

Nowag B., Casabona G., Kippenberger S. et al. Calcium hydroxylapatite microspheres activate fibroblasts through direct contact to stimulate neocollagenesis. J Cosmet Dermatol 2023; 22(2): 426–432.

Obregon M.J. Changing white into brite adipocytes. Focus on "BMP4 and BMP7 induce the white-to-brown transition of primary human adipose stem cells." Am J Physiol Cell Physiol 2014; 306(5): 425–427.

Oliveira S.M.D., Rocha L.B., da Cunha M.T.R. et al. Effects of carboxytherapy on skin laxity. J Cosmet Dermatol 2020; 19(11): 3007–3013.

Omi T., Sato S., Kawana S. Ultrastructural assessment of cellulite morphology: clues to a therapeutic strategy? Laser Ther 2013; 22(2): 131–136.

Ou M.Y., Zhang H., Tan P.C. et al. Adipose tissue aging: mechanisms and therapeutic implications. Cell Death Dis 2022; 13(4): 300.

Pacifico M., Kanapathy M., Dancey A. et al. Summary document on safety and recommendations for aesthetic liposuction: Joint British Association of Aesthetic Plastic Surgeons (BAAPS)/British Association of Plastic Reconstructive and Aesthetic Surgeons (BAPRAS) expert liposuction group. J Plast Reconstr Aesthet Surg 2022; 75(3): 941–947.

Papafotiou C., Christaki E., van den Akker E.L. et al. Hair cortisol concentrations exhibit a positive association with salivary cortisol profiles and are increased in obese prepubertal girls. Stress 2017; 20(2): 217–222.

Park S.Y., Kim S.B., Wan J. et al. Lipolytic agents for submental fat reduction: Review. Skin Res Technol 2024; 30(2): e13601.

Parpaite T., Coste B. Piezo channels. Current Biol 2017; 27(7): R243–R258.

Peng Y., Zhao L., Li M. et al. Plasticity of adipose tissues: interconversion among white, brown, and beige fat and its role in energy homeostasis. Biomolecules 2024; 14(4): 483.

Pera F., Suman C., Cosma M. et al. Intertrigo in severe obesity: clinical insights and outcomes with a new antimicrobial silver-infused breathable fabric. J Cosmet Dermatol 2025; 24(5): e70161.

Peterkova V.A., Vasyukova O.V. On the issue of a new classification of obesity in children and adolescents. Prob Endocrinol 2015; 2: 39–44.

Pfisterer K., Shaw L.E., Symmank D., Weninger W. The Extracellular matrix in skin inflammation and infection. Front Cell Dev Biol 2021; 9: 682414.

Piccolo D., Mutlag M.H., Fusco I., Bonan P. Facial and body contouring with 1444 nm Nd:YAG laser-assisted lipolysis: Clinical evidence. Skin Res Technol 2023; 29(7): e13400.

Piddini E. Epithelial homeostasis: a Piezo of the puzzle. Curr Biol 2017; 27(6): R232–R234.

Pilch W., Czerwińska-Ledwig O., Chitryniewicz-Rostek J. et al. The impact of vibration therapy interventions on skin condition and skin temperature changes in young women with lipodystrophy: a pilot study. Evid Based Complement Alternat Med 2019; 2019: 8436325.

Pina-Vidal C., Berned-Samatán V., Piera E. et al. Mechanochemical encapsulation of caffeine in UIO-66 and UIO-66-NH2 to obtain polymeric composites by extrusion with recycled polyamide 6 or polylactic acid biopolymer. Polymers (Basel). 2024; 16(5): 637.

Pinto H., Melamed G. Contrast lipocryolysis: preand post-session tempering improves clinical results. Adipocyte 2014; 3(3): 212–214.

Pinto H.R., Garcia-Cruz E., Melamed G.E. A study to evaluate the action of lipocryolysis. Cryo Letters 2012; 33(3): 177–181.

Pitche P., Diatta B., Faye O. et al. Risk factors associated with leg erysipelas (cellulitis) in sub-Saharan Africa: a multicentre case-control study [French]. Ann Dermatol Venereol 2015; 142(11): 633–638.

Pollard T.D. Actin and actin-binding proteins. Cold Spring Harb Perspect Biol 2016; 8: a018226.

Pollard T.D., Goldman R.D. Overview of the cytoskeleton from an evolutionary perspective. Cold Spring Harb Perspect Biol 2018; 10(7): a030288.

Ptaszek B., Wójciak A., Żak A., Podsiadło S. The effect of lower limb pressotherapy treatment on selected rheological and biochemical indices of blood in young, healthy women. J Clin Med 2024; 13(19): 5743.

Pumprla J., Howorka K., Kolackova Z., Sovova E. Non-contact radiofrequency-induced reduction of subcutaneous abdominal fat correlates with initial cardiovascular autonomic balance and fat tissue hormones: safety analysis. F1000Res 2015; 4: 49.

Qiu J., Yue F., Zhu P. et al. FAM210A is essential for cold-induced mitochondrial remodeling in brown adipocytes. Nat Commun 2023; 14(1): 6344.

Quesada-Cortés A., Campos-Muñoz L., Díaz-Díaz R.M. et al. Cold panniculitis. Dermatol Clin 2008; 26: 485–489, vii.

Ridone P., Vassalli M., Martinac B. Piezo1 mechanosensitive channels: what are they and why are they important. Biophys Rev 2019; 11(5): 795-805.

Rose P.T., Morgan M. Histological changes associated with mesotherapy for fat dissolution. J Cosmet Laser Ther 2005; 7(1): 17–19.

Rosen J., Darwin E., Tuchayi S.M. et al. Skin changes and manifestations associated with the treatment of obesity. J Am Acad Dermatol 2019; 81(5): 1059–1069.

Rotunda A.M., Kolodney M.S. Mesotherapy and phosphatidylcholine injections: historical clarification and review. Dermatol Surg 2006; 32(4): 465–480.

Rotunda A.M., Suzuki H., Moy R.T. et al. Detergent effects of sodium deoxycholate are a major feature of an injectable phosphatidylcholine formulation used for localized fat dissolution. Dermatol Surg 2004; 30(7): 1001–1008.

Royo de la Torre J., Moreno-Moraga J., Muñoz E., Cornejo Navarro P. Multisource, phase-controlled radiofrequency for treatment of skin laxity: correlation between clinical and in-vivo confocal microscopy results and real-time thermal changes. J Clin Aesthet Dermatol 2011; 4(1): 28–35.

Sadala A.Y., Rampazo É.P., Liebano R.E. Vibration anesthesia during carboxytherapy for cellulite: a study protocol. Pain Manag 2022; 12(4): 401–408.

Sakers A., De Siqueira M.K., Seale P., Villanueva C.J. Adipose-tissue plasticity in health and disease. Cell 2022; 185(3): 419–446.

Sakon M., Ariyoshi H., Umeshita K., Monden M. Ischemia-reperfusion injury of the liver with special reference to calcium-dependent mechanisms. Surg Today 2002; 32(1): 1–12.

Salti G., Ghersetich I,. Tantussi F. et al. Phosphatidylcholine and sodium deoxycholate in the treatment of localized fat: a double-blind, randomized study. Dermatol Surg 2008; 34(1): 60–66.

Saponaro C., Gaggini M., Carli F., Gastaldelli A. The subtle balance between lipolysis and lipogenesis: a critical point in metabolic homeostasis. Nutrients 2015; 7(11): 9453–9474.

Sasaki G.H., Abelev N., Tevez-Ortiz A. Noninvasive selective cryolipolysis and reperfusion recovery for localized natural fat reduction and contouring. Aesthet Surg J 2014; 34(3): 420–431.

Savacini M.B., Bueno D.T., Molina A.C.S. et al. Effectiveness and safety of contrast cryolipolysis for subcutaneous-fat reduction. Dermatol Res Pract 2018; 2018: 5276528.

Savoia A., Landi S., Vannini F., Baldi A. Low-level laser therapy and vibration therapy for the treatment of localized adiposity and fibrous cellulite. Dermatol Ther 2013; 3(1): 41–52.

Schilling L., Saedi N., Weiss R. 1060 nm diode hyperthermic laser lipolysis: the latest in non-invasive body contouring. J Drugs Dermatol 2017; 16(1): 48–52.

Seaman S.A., Tannan S.C., Cao Y. et al. Paradoxical adipose hyperplasia and cellular effects after cryolipolysis: a case report. Aesthet Surg J 2016; 36(1): NP6–13.

Sebo Z.L., Rodeheffer M.S. Assembling the adipose organ: adipocyte lineage segregation and adipogenesis in vivo. Development 2019; 146(7): dev172098.

Sergeev I.N., Aljutaily T., Walton G., Huarte E. Effects of synbiotic supplement on human gut microbiota, body composition and weight loss in obesity. Nutrients 2020; 12(1): 222.

Severinsen M.C.K., Pedersen B.K. Muscle-organ crosstalk: the emerging roles of myokines. Endocr Rev 2020; 41(4): 594–609.

Shareef L.G., Khalid S.S., Raheem M.F. et al. Population-level interest in glucagon-like peptide-1 receptor agonists for weight loss using Google Trends statistics in a 12-month retrospective analysis: an infodemiology and infoveillance study. Cureus 2024; 16(10): e71569.

Shek S.Y., Chan N.P., Chan H.H. Non-invasive cryolipolysis for body contouring in Chinese: A first commercial experience. Lasers Surg Med 2012; 44(2): 125–130.

Shipman A.R., Millington G.W. Obesity and the skin. Br J Dermatol 2011; 165(4): 743–750.

Shridharani S.M., Broyles J.M., Matarasso A. Liposuction devices: technology update. Med Devices (Auckl) 2014; 7: 241–251.

Siems W., Grune T., Voss P., Brenke R. Anti-fibrosclerotic effects of shock wave therapy in lipedema and cellulite. BioFactors 2005; 24(1–4): 275–282.

Silva G.A.T., Souza D.R., Parreiras K.E.C. et al. Effectiveness of cryolipolysis for subcutaneous fat reduction: a systematic review and meta-analysis. Surg Cosmet Dermatol 2021;13: e20210004.

Singh S.M., Geddes E.R., Boutrous S.G. et al. Paradoxical adipose hyperplasia secondary to cryolipolysis: an underreported entity? Lasers Surg Med 2015; 47(6): 476–478.

Song T., Kuang S. Adipocyte dedifferentiation in health and diseases. Clin Sci (Lond) 2019; 133(20): 2107–2119.

Stefani W.A. Adipose hypertrophy following cryolipolysis. Aesthet Surg J 2015; 35(7): 218–20.

Steinberg D. Hormonal control of lipolysis in adipose tissue. Adv Exp Med Biol 1972; 26(0): 77–88.

Stevens W.G., Bachelor E.P. Cryolipolysis conformable-surface applicator for non-surgical fat reduction in lateral thighs. Aesthet Surg J 2015; 35(1): 66–71.

Stroumza N., Gauthier N., Senet P., et al. Paradoxical adipose hypertrophy (PAH) after cryolipolysis. Aesthet Surg J 2018; 38(4): 411–417.

Surowiecka A., Strużyna J. Adipose-derived stem cells for facial rejuvenation. J Pers Med 2022; 12(1): 117.

Susini P., di Seclì D., Bacchini S. et al. Carboxytherapy in dermatologic surgery and aesthetic medicine: current knowledge and future perspectives-a systematic review. Dermatol Surg 2025; 51(7): 673–678.

Taira K.G., Wang M., Guo W. et al. Association of cellulitis with obesity: systematic review and meta-analysis. JMIR Dermatol. 2024; 7: e54302.

Tan H.C., Dampil O.A., Marquez M.M. Efficacy and safety of semaglutide for weight loss in obesity without diabetes: a systematic review and meta-analysis. J ASEAN Fed Endocr Soc 2022; 37(2): 65–72.

Tao L., Yi Y. Recombinant type III humanized collagen solution for injection improves skin photoaging in Chinese population: a case series. J Cosmet Dermatol 2025; 24(7): e70276.

Tchernof A., Després J.P. Sex steroid hormones, sex hormone-binding globulin, and obesity in men and women. Horm Metab Res 2000; 32(11–12): 526–536.

Theodorou S.J., Del Vecchio D., Chia C.T. Soft tissue contraction in body contouring with radiofrequency-assisted liposuction: a treatment gap solution. Aesthet Surg J 2018; 38(Suppl 2): S74–S83.

Troia S., Moreira A.M., Pisco D. et al. Effect of shock wave therapy associated with aerobic exercise on cellulite: A randomized controlled trial. J Cosmet Dermatol 2021; 20(6): 1732–1742.

Vecchia P., Matthes R., Ziegelberger G., et al. Exposure to high frequency electromagnetic fields, biological effects and health consequences (100 kHz-300 GHz). International Commission on Non-Ionizing Radiation Protection, 2009.

Verner I. A novel nonfocused pulsed ultrasound technology for noninvasive circumference reduction. Dermatol Ther 2021; 34(5): e15101.

Villagrasa-Boli P., Monte-Serrano J., Álvarez-Salafranca M. et al. Obesity-associated lymphedematous mucinosis: dermoscopic-histopathological findings and differential diagnosis. Int J Dermatol 2022; 61(8): e304–e306.

Vivas A., Lev-Tov H., Kirsner R.S. Venous leg ulcers. Ann Intern Med 2016; 165(3): ITC17–ITC32.

Vostrikova A.V. Electromyostimulation — a new direction in aesthetic body contour correction with unique possibilities. Cosmetics & Medicine 2022; 1: 66–75.

Watanabe M., Risi R., Masi D. et al. Current evidence to propose different food supplements for weight loss: a comprehensive review. Nutrients 2020; 12(9): 2873.

Weiss R.A., Bernardy J. Induction of fat apoptosis by a non-thermal device: mechanism of action of non-invasive high-intensity electromagnetic technology in a porcine model. Lasers Surg Med 2019; 51(1): 47–53.

Wigley C.H., Janssen T.J., Mosahebi A. Shock wave therapy in plastic surgery: a review of the current indications. Aesthet Surg J 2023; 43(3): 370–386.

Wu J., Cohen P., Spiegelman B.M. Adaptive thermogenesis in adipocytes: is beige the new brown? Genes Dev 2013; 27(3): 234–250.

Wu S., Coombs D.M., Gurunian R. Liposuction: concepts, safety, and techniques in body contouring surgery. Cleve Clin J Med 2020; 87(6): 367–375.

Youngstrom T.G., Bartness T.J. White adipose tissue sympathetic nervous system denervation increases fat pad mass and fat cell number. Am J Physiol 1998; 275(5): R1488–1493.

Zaccaron R.P., Mendes C., da Costa C. et al. Skin metabolism in obesity: a narrative review. Wound Repair Regen 2024; 32(6): 1022–1027.

Zelickson B., Egbert B.M., Preciado J. et al. Cryolipolysis for noninvasive fat cell destruction: initial results from a pig model. Dermatol Surg 2009. 35(10): 1462–1470.

Zelickson B.D., Burns A.J., Kilmer S.L. Cryolipolysis for safe and effective inner thigh fat reduction. Lasers Surg Med 2015; 47(2): 120–127.

Zhang A., Silverberg J. Association of atopic dermatitis with being overweight and obese: a systematic review and meta-analysis. J Am Acad Dermatol 2015; 72(4): 606–616.

Zinngrebe J., Debatin K.M., Fischer-Posovszky P. Adipocytes in hematopoiesis and acute leukemia: friends, enemies, or innocent bystanders? Leukemia 2020; 34(9): 2305–2316.

Zornoza B., Rubio C., Piera E. et al. Caffeine encapsulation in metal organic framework MIL-53(Al) at pilot plant scale for preparation of polyamide textile fibers with cosmetic properties. ACS Appl Mater Interfaces 2022; 14(19): 22476–22488.